I0765194

Two Chai Day

ONE WIDOW'S STORY ABOUT LIVING BEYOND GRIEF

IRENE McGOLDRICK, MSW

iUniverse, Inc.
Bloomington

Two Chai Day
One Widow's Story about Living beyond Grief

iUniverse Star
an iUniverse, Inc. imprint

iUniverse books may be ordered through booksellers or by contacting:

iUniverse
1663 Liberty Drive
Bloomington, IN 47403
www.iuniverse.com
1-800-Authors (1-800-288-4677)

Because of the dynamic nature of the Internet, any Web addresses or links contained in this book may have changed since publication and may no longer be valid. The views expressed in this work are solely those of the author and do not necessarily reflect the views of the publisher, and the publisher hereby disclaims any responsibility for them.

ISBN: 978-1-936236-79-4 (sc)
ISBN: 978-1-936236-80-0 (e)

Library of Congress Control Number: 2011913705

Printed in the United States of America

iUniverse rev. date: 7/29/2011

Author's Note

Woven into the story you are about to read are selected entries from my late husband's personal journals. They are his uncensored thoughts. Using them in this story was not an easy decision. His journals were not something he shared with me when he was alive and, in fact, caused some friction at times. So I do not open them to the public lightly.

I couldn't ask him, obviously, but when I imagined asking him, I could clearly hear Bob saying to me, "Renie, I'm dead. Do what you want."

His journals provide a unique opportunity for me to use his words. Through his journals, we are able to write our story together. I truly feel that his words are a gift he left not only for his children and me, but for anyone who might benefit from reading them.

I know he would be proud to know that his struggles could help someone in a similar situation. Isn't that what we all want?

DEDICATION

For Bob - the undead dad - You will always be alive in our hearts.
—Love, Henry, Arthur and Irene

We Remain Upright

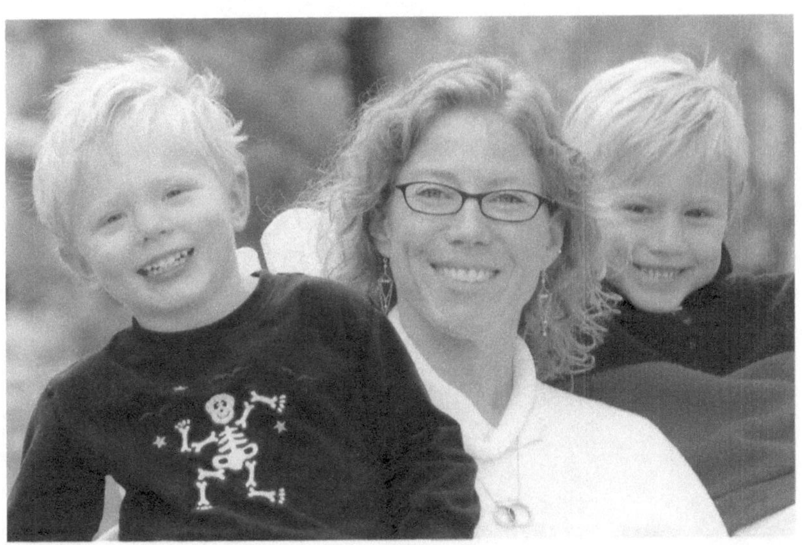

It's not having what you want
it's wanting what you've got.
Sheryl Crow, *Soak Up the Sun*

Arthur and I were in the car and waiting for Henry to get out of his kindergarten class. The minivans and SUVs were lined up obediently. Henry was ushered out of the brick building. With his eyes toward the ground, he nodded almost imperceptibly to the teacher as she complimented him on his hard work for the day. He got in the car, placed his canvas school bag on the seat next to him, buckled himself up, and leaned over to his brother.

"Arthur, when are you going to start using the toilet?" he asked.

"When my daddy gets back," Arthur answered.

"Arthur, Daddy's dead. It makes us all sad. And I still cry about it sometimes, but he's on Dog Mountain now. And also in the dining room—in that thing on the shelf—you know. So he isn't coming back, Arthur. But you still have to use the toilet."

Arthur answered simply, "I know, Henry."

I glanced in the rearview mirror and saw two blonde heads leaning toward each other. Both sets of blue eyes gazed out their own windows. Henry sounded so serious and thoughtful, as if he had been thinking about the conversation for days and had chosen his words carefully, just as his dad once had.

At the time Henry shared this straightforward bit of advice with his younger brother, he was six years old. Arthur was three, and their dad had been dead almost three years.

Their dad, my husband, died early in the morning on March 29, 2004.

This is our story.

Chapter One

The Forest and the Trees

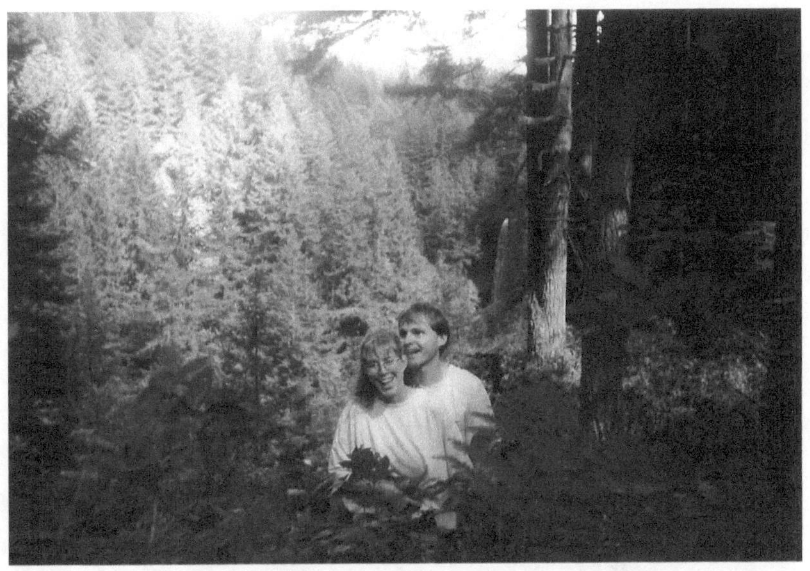

Lovers don't finally meet somewhere.
They're in each other all along.
Mawlana Jalal-al-Din Rumi

I had a premonition.

It was early in the fall of 2002.

It was *before*.

Just out of the shower, I stood on the second floor landing of our big old four-square home and watched Bob whisper good-night to Henry. The steam from the bathroom followed me, curling my damp hair and bringing with it the smell of peppermint and rosemary. Bob was on his knees, leaning over Henry as he lay in his bed. I could see the dark pupils of Henry's eyes as he concentrated on Bob. Henry looked so small in his new "big boy bed". He had just turned two.

The bright colors of the helicopters and dump trucks on Henry's new quilt jumped out against the freshly painted blue walls. The two messy blonde heads touched each other lightly as they plotted the possibilities of what Henry could dream about that night.

Unable to take my eyes off this idyllic scene, I slowly became aware of warm breath in my ear, as if someone whispered to me. I cocked my head towards the familiar-sounding voice.

"Remember this moment, remember right now." The words seeped into my consciousness like a slow, rolling fog.

I felt a breeze move just beneath my skin, raising the hair on my arms, and a slight tingle on my scalp. It seemed a long-forgotten secret, embedded in my cells long ago, was pulled to the surface by this vision in front of me. The sensation felt like a word on the tip of my tongue or an interrupted thought I couldn't recall.

"*This won't last,*" I was warned by a voice from the dark recesses of my mind, the primitive part that doesn't think in words as much as in basic emotions.

Immediately I made a mental picture of the two of them in the bedroom with their heads together and stored it away in my mind. Being a planner, I figured I should keep the tableau safe in my mind, just in case.

The secret left as quickly as it came, leaving my limbs feeling stiff, as if the memory did not want to be too far away from the surface.

≈≈

I take great pride in following through with my plans. I planned on finishing college in Colorado and traveling in Europe with girlfriends, and I did. I planned on moving back to the Midwest to work and finish graduate school, and I did. I planned on moving to a different city to start my career after completing my MSW, and I did. I planned on never getting married and never having kids.

I didn't plan on Bob.

≈≈

We met in the dank employee break room at Great Harvest Bread Company in Whitefish Bay, Wisconsin. I sat at the table and watched Bob from underneath my dirty Cubs baseball cap as he talked to some coworkers about a camping trip he was planning. Butter and honey dripped on my hands from the warm bread I held.

Something about his almost slouching, relaxed posture and the subtle movements of his slender fingers while he spoke seemed so familiar. His tone was easy and his words precise.

Oh, there you are. I thought to myself.

I had never seen him before, but I felt as if we had planned to meet in that cool basement that day. As if the camping trip he was planning was already on my calendar—Camping w/Bob—had been marked on the square for September 18, 1993.

Never mind I didn't own a sleeping bag; I was going on that camping trip.

≈≈

Fast-forward nine years.

We were back in the Midwest after a four-year sojourn in Portland, Oregon. Where better to fall in love than there among the lush green ferns, enormous Douglas firs, and clean, moist air of the Pacific Northwest?

We were married and living in a big, old house with a son. Bob was teaching high school science, and I was a social worker at an adult day center.

Where did all this domesticity come from?

Ah, yes, the Bob-and-Irene plan, the plan that we two hatched while hiking on trails blanketed by pine needles and the occasional banana slug. This plan involved working and raising our son, maybe having another one; it involved camping and hiking and biking and traveling.

Our plan never included a cancer diagnosis at thirty-eight.

That was never part of the plan.

Plans change.

≈≈

In the fall of 2002, we had been back in Milwaukee for almost three years, and our son, Henry, was two. Bob started complaining of shoulder pain. He had some theories regarding the stress involved with his teaching job and body mechanics. He made some adjustments, and life went on. The pain did not go away, however. He became increasingly frustrated and depressed and began to write in his journal more.

The depression did not alarm us initially because Bob had what I referred to as "a depression cycle". In fact, we blamed the entire situation on his depression and prepared ourselves for another "bad period". These "bad periods" were not all that bad for me; he didn't sleep all the time or withdraw from the family as you might imagine. I usually noticed an increase in his journaling activity. During these times Bob would also increase his physical activity, so these periods also meant more bike riding and jaunts to the park.

Bob had started writing a journal in high school, trying to make sense of his anger and angst at that time and finding release and solace in his written thoughts.

Bob's journal entry
October 20, 2002

I write because I am afraid of loss. I write because I have nowhere to go. I write because I am trying to expunge anger and sadness. I write because I am trying to reveal joy and understanding. I write because I like seeing miracles appear on the page. I write because there is no one listening. I write because I'm angry. I write because I am sad. I write because I am ecstatic. I write because I am in awe. I write because I do not understand. I write to feed whatever glowing embers are in my mind. I write to see my mind. I write to find my mind. I write to ask, "What is my mind?" I write to realize how little I know and how much. I write because I like to draw. I write because I think there is value in this mess of head voices.

In the beginning of our relationship, we might have been derailed by Bob's depression. Not keeping a journal myself, I was perturbed by the feeling of secrecy surrounding the notebook.

I would pester him about it. "Why can't you talk to me about it? Maybe I can help. You can tell me anything."

Bob had already shared his biggest secret with me very early in our relationship. We were sitting on a picnic table down by Lake Michigan, breathing in the early fall air, and its scent of dry leaves, and the slightly fishy smell of the lake. It is easy to be open when it's dark and you can hear the calming waves steadily rolling in and out. We were busy having the kind of conversation that a new couple has, sharing stories of our childhoods, our family lore, our college antics.

Bob shared the information that he had been molested by the family barber as a child. As he shared this very personal information with me, he was very matter-of-fact and sounded somewhat detached from the words, as if they were floating above him and not actually coming out of his mouth. Bob explained that between the ages of seven and about ten, his dad would drop him off at the barber's shop, leave, and run some errands while Bob got his hair cut.

When Bob was a child, most people trusted others far more readily than they do now. Bob's dad, Hank, a wiry, industrious, no-nonsense guy, never thought for a minute that he was putting his son in any danger. And Bob never told his dad or anyone in his family about the molestation at the time.

But he wrote about it in his journals. When Bob hit puberty and the gravity of the crime began to enter his consciousness, he became confused about his own role in the events. He blamed his dad for putting him in the situation that allowed them to happen. His was a rational thought process for a confused and angry teenager.

By the time we met, Bob had done lots of talk therapy and reading. He tried to resolve the uncertainties these events of his childhood left for him as an adult. He tried to settle the troubling feelings of shame and guilt that the molestation elicited and the anger and silence that had arisen between him and his father as he became a young adult. He kept writing in his journals.

A few months before Bob and I met, he had read about his molester's death in the obituaries. Bob had just returned to Milwaukee from Atlanta and was living back in the same neighborhood where the crime occurred. As if drawn by a magnet and concurrently repelled by some opposing force, Bob always returned to Milwaukee after trying out a different state to call home for a while.

The news of his molester's death had sent Bob into a relapse.

Bob's journal entry
April 10/11, 1993

There is sadness and anger always in my eyes and voice. I can hardly imagine sincere and pleasant laughter, especially now with the quiet and the rain. I seem so detached from the events and people around me. I look for people I can help, for this seems to be my only worth. I know, though, that I have the capacity to be interesting and pleasant. I crave this silence, though, now. It frightens me in a comforting way.

I don't know if I hold unrealistic expectations of myself. I want everyone to love me, I want to have deep meaningful relationships, I want to feel proud of who I am and what I do. I want to feel surrounded by people who love and care about me. I want to live a life of high adventure.

It seems though as if this day will pass in more silence. Silence, silence, silence. I am now the enforcer of my silence. The mantle has been passed, and I have accepted it, reluctantly and with seemingly little choice. The passing, though, may have been slow and unnoticed, and I may, only now, be becoming aware of my crucial role.

I feel as if my soul is withering and dying in this silence.

≈≈

Being nosy and more than a bit worried about how I would handle this situation over the long haul, I even stole a peek at a journal once. I confessed shortly afterwards, not being able to stand myself. Bob was very level-headed, realistic, and disappointed. I was so sorry. I thought he should leave me. I felt awful about what I had done and even worse about what I had read. I hoped I hadn't ruined his trust. I hoped I had enough self-confidence to trust him now, to believe the feelings he voiced. They were sometimes different from the ones he wrote.

The experience made me examine my own head voices. I did not yet understand that we all have thoughts that we keep to ourselves. Some people write these thoughts down on paper. It is a brave thing to do. It can actually be frightening to see the alter ego express itself in written words, for such words are proof of its existence.

This is the card Bob wrote to me the day after my confession.

Spring 1994
Renie,

I don't know what I did to deserve you. In fact, I don't think I could have done anything to deserve you. You are just one of those incredible fortunate events that happen to grace the face of this planet, and I happen to be the lucky one to share your world.

I once read that being in love does not consist of gazing into each other's eyes but of looking out in the same direction together. I feel this is true and that I am truly in love with you.

I've met all sorts of wonderful people in my life, Renie, but I have never met anyone like you, and I can't imagine that I ever will. When I think of you, all I imagine is kindness and strength and honesty and, of course raw, unabashed, passionate sexuality and umpteen other wonderful qualities that all add up to this wonderfully lovely humanness. Anyway, I think you are pretty cool.

I don't mean to keep any part of myself from you, Renie, it's just that I seem to have spent a lot of time learning the fine art of talking myself into a hole. There's no mystery or tragedy to it. It's just a dumb trick that, at one time, may have been more helpful than it is now, but it's just an unnecessary habit that doesn't do me any good. So if I seem to

deemphasize it, it's not because I don't want to share something with you … .well, okay, it's because I don't want to share something with you. I guess I'm still confused about this. It's like having a limp that resulted from an injury that is mostly healed, but I just fall into from time to time by force of habit. I'm ashamed of this habit, but I also fear that if you see me limping, then this will make you start limping too, and then I will be responsible for your limp. I don't know. Anyway, I LOVE YOU,
Bob

And with that, I was free!

Everyone is responsible for his or her own happiness. This is the best lesson Bob ever taught me and the cornerstone of our relationship. Bob wanted to be with me, but he did not need me. Frankly, I didn't really want all that responsibility anyway. I couldn't have taken that on and wouldn't have wanted to risk feeling burdened. We didn't need to hold each other's hands, but we knew we had each other's backs.

≈≈

As the winter of 2003 progressed, Bob's health began to spiral downward with a series of odd, seemingly unrelated issues. First, the pain in his shoulder spread to his knee and turned severe. One cold Saturday afternoon, Henry and I were playing at the bottom of the stairs. The sun shone through the stained glass windows in our foyer, making small dusty rainbows that floated in the air.

Henry liked to pile his blocks on the patches of red, yellow and green that filtered through the pocket door and landed on the tan carpet. He was fascinated by the way the reflections changed the color of the wood in his hands.

Bob was in the pantry, rearranging our dwindling stock of canned peaches and pears, methodically moving the Ball jars from one side of the pantry to the other. I could hear the clinking of the glass as Bob lined the jars up next to one another. He had the phone balanced between his shoulder and cheek as he told the on-call nurse about the pain he was experiencing, explaining to her that he had taken some Vicodin he had left over from some earlier situation.

I suddenly felt uneasy. *My God, what's going on? He sounds like a junkie on the phone. Are we in trouble here?*

≈≈

On January 30, not long after that phone conversation, Bob and I were in bed. My hand slowly moved down his spine towards the gentle curve at the base.

"Shit, Bob, what is that?" I yelled as I sat up abruptly. My hand had settled on a mass about the size of a half dollar.

Then the lights came on. Henry was making his way up the stairs to our room, quickly, on his two-year-old legs.

"Shit," we both whispered in unison as his little blonde head and those serious blue eyes emerged over the ridge of the top step.

Once Henry was settled back in under his comforter, his head poking out from under the helicopters and trucks of its print, I returned to our room.

The romance of earlier was over the instant my hand felt that mass. I was all business now.

"You have to go to the doctor *tomorrow*! Promise me! What the hell is that? That thing cannot be good!" My voice was high with concern, and my heart began to pulse rapidly.

"I'll call," Bob responded, yawning.

"Tomorrow! You're going tomorrow," I insisted.

"Tomorrow, Renie. I'll go tomorrow."

≈≈

He was told it was a cyst.

"Cysts come and go," the doctor said. "Keep an eye on it."

Bob immediately took himself off the Zoloft he had started a few months earlier when the depression had first crept up on him. He had never taken medication to deal with his depression, preferring to work it out on the pages of his journal and by using a book titled *Feeling Good*, by David Burns, that he found particularly helpful.

He had been doing some Internet research and had read in a chat room that some people on Zoloft had developed cysts. I don't know if this suspected side effect was grounded in anything other than confusion on Bob's part.

Bob was trying to connect the dots, to gather information like the scientist he was, and all he came up with was a jumble of lines leading nowhere.

≈≈

Bob's journal entry
February 24, 2003

Irene is pregnant. She did the test yesterday. She thinks we're going to have a girl. I came close to scheduling a vasectomy last summer. I never got around to it, but I was pretty serious about doing it. I was pretty surprised when Irene made the shift to wanting another child. I never really imagined she would. I know that I felt a certain tinge of sadness for Henry, being an only child. I think I had reconciled myself to it, though, and I was becoming more appreciative of the simplicity of having only one child.

That's all history, though. Now we just have to hang on for the ride. I love the idea of having another child. It's an amazing rush, exciting, mysterious. I get to see Irene pregnant again; we get to see another little person join the world.

≈≈

We planned this pregnancy, and the baby followed the plan perfectly. That child took his one shot to enter into this world. One month earlier, we were not trying yet; one month later, and Bob was in the hospital. After that, we would have never tried again. Call the force behind these events fate, call it luck, or call it God. Call it the cosmic universe and those cosmic deals that are made before entering this incarnation. Call it craziness.

The idea of a second pregnancy had come up suddenly. I knew it was not the most practical choice at the time, and I tried to make sure the urge wasn't just a fleeting impulse. One weekend when we were in the height of the baby debate, we were at a hotel with our friends, Jeanne and Jim, attempting to escape the desolate winter.

Jeanne and Jim were my first friends in Milwaukee. Jeanne was a pragmatic journalist. She had the kind of ivory complexion and silky hair I associate with the female characters in Jane Austen's novels. She was a perfect match to my sarcastic humor and had an equal love for talking endlessly about other people's lives. Jim was a photographer, thin and pale, with a look in his eyes that told me he saw more through his lens than one might care to know. Jim once took apart a pair of new tennis shoes, layer by layer, because they squeaked when he walked. Bob and I showed up at their house one evening, and the destroyed shoes were strewn about the side steps.

The three of us met through a mutual friend, though none of us were crazy about him. However, we three really liked each other. I ditched the guy (his black leather pants and gun-toting tool belt should have been reasons enough), and the three of us became inseparable. Luckily, when Bob entered the picture, we formed a good foursome. Bob's observant style fit well with Jim's solemn nature, and the boys often wandered off to sit in silence while we girls chatted.

Jeanne and I were in the pool entertaining the kids that night, and we both watched as Bob ambled across the room to get in the hot tub. He was holding his right arm at the elbow, trying to alleviate some of the pain in his shoulder as he limped by us.

"What's that thing on Bob's back?" Jeanne asked, wrinkling her nose.

"It's a cyst, according to the doctor," I told her, trying to sound convincing. I felt self-conscious for Bob. The cyst was so unsightly.

"You don't sound so sure," she responded.

"Something's just not right with him. I'm wondering if now is really the right time to be trying to get pregnant." I cautiously waited for her response. The smell of chlorine filled the air around us.

"What do you mean?"

"I just don't think we should be getting pregnant when Bob could have spinal cancer or something." I was attempting to be dramatic to lessen the impact of my very real concern.

"Oh, he doesn't have spinal cancer," Jeanne answered, right on cue.

Bob and I did not get pregnant accidentally or carelessly; the pregnancy was a careful, considered choice. Were we blind to what was right in front of us? Were we in denial? Was the idea of having a baby some kind of subconscious effort to bring life and hope into our house? Was a baby a distraction? All those motivations were in play, I suppose. Whatever it was, we got pregnant in the midst of all the craziness and gloom.

Being pregnant and having your husband treated for cancer is not a combination of events I could have ever planned.

Arthur had his own plans.

≈≈

Bob's journal entry
March 9, 2003

I have gum disease. I need a root canal. I'm going to have two teeth removed for sure, possibly four, and I also need gum surgery. And I'm in pain. I want all this shit done right now. I've been thinking this was a sinus infection for about two months now. I went through finding out I was allergic to Amoxicillin, which I was taking for the probably nonexistent sinus infection and now I might have to wait a month and a half to get this surgery. I've been taking Vicodin nightly because that's when the pain really kicks in. I take it along with a Benadryl to knock me out. Last night it didn't work too well, but the night before I slept pretty good. Tonight isn't looking too good, though.

My health for the last six months has been a concern for both Irene and I. I've had this chronic knee pain that seems to have gone away. I've had this pain and swelling in my right shoulder, and this is still a problem. I also have several cysts, one on my lower back, one above my ear and one on my right arm. And along with all of this the goddamn tooth pain, which is really the focus of my attention now.

≈≈

Henry was always an early riser, and I mean *early*. I once told Bob's family that if Henry ever slept until 7:00 AM, I would swim naked in Lake Michigan. That was how unlikely the prospect sounded to me.

I, on the other hand, am not a morning person. To say I am not a morning person is like saying childbirth kind of hurts or that the polar ice caps are melting is a bit of a concern. OK, so that might be a little dramatic, but I really don't like to get out of bed in the morning.

Once Henry had learned to get out of the crib that once contained him and roam freely in the house, I would wake up to feel him literally dragging me out of bed, saying, "I want to see your feet.". I would poke my feet out from beneath the covers, my dishwater blonde hair a tangled mess on top of my head, and wiggle them around for him. This was my desperate attempt to stay horizontal just one more minute.

"On the floor," Henry would say.

One memorable February morning it wasn't Henry who woke me, but Bob, looming over me in the darkness. My nose was cold, and I pulled the down comforter up and tucked it under my chin. Our room was on the third floor. It was a converted attic space with no direct heat source and became rather icy in the winter. I tried to focus on Bob through my early morning haze. He was rubbing his arms up and down with his hands, thrusting them out toward me with a look of disbelief and dismay.

"Renie, I have to go the ER. Man, I think I have the chicken pox or something," he said, incredulous.

I burst out laughing. It was one of those completely inappropriate emotional responses to information. The appropriate response would be concern, of course, or possibly an offer of a ride to the hospital.

But I laughed. I laughed, and Bob left, taking himself to the ER. As for myself, I rolled over, pulled the feather comforter over my head, buried my head in the figurative sand, and went back to sleep. I woke up a bit later when Henry pulled me out of bed, demanding his morning smoothie.

The mind protects us from information it is not ready to process. But the body knows. That cold February morning, I knew something was terribly wrong with Bob, but I was terrified of thinking or, God forbid, speaking these concerns—then I would have to act on them. It would make them real and not just the rumination of an overactive imagination. I would have to admit Bob was sick and then deal with what all that sickness might mean. I didn't want to go down that path. Not then, not yet.

So when Bob showed up at the bedside that morning, with concern and obvious discomfort on his face, I had to laugh. His full-body rash was no laughing matter, but I had to laugh. I was too afraid to cry. I was hardly even surprised by the news. I mean, why not?

"Why not chicken pox?" I blathered to my girlfriends at play group later that day. The bedroom was filled with the activities of our two-year olds, little teacups and plastic plates, wooden moons that balanced on their sides. "Muscle pain," I continued, "cysts, growths, oral surgery, sinus infection, rashes. Of course, chicken pox." The tears standing in my eyes defied my attempt at humor. I felt on the verge of hysteria; that tightrope between reason and insanity is sometimes just a matter of context.

"I'm sure he's fine, Irene. It's been a long winter for all of us," one of my friends said. They all looked at me quizzically.

These women had all undergone natural child birth and were not easily spooked. I could see in their eyes that they didn't understand my fears, but they weren't living in my house. They didn't know that Bob hadn't slept in our bed for weeks because he had been forced to sleep sitting up in a chair to avoid the pain that lying down caused. They didn't know that cysts were cropping up in new places on his body overnight. They didn't smell the sharp scent of fear that I picked up the minute I entered our house, a scent so thick that it infected every thought we had and made even the smallest task of daily living seem monumental.

≈≈

Now I was crying, the tears silently leaking from my eyes. The nervous laughter of the other morning had progressed to true fear. "Bob, I'm really worried. I'm scared there's something really wrong with you."

We were sitting next to each other on the edge of the guest bed. It had only been a couple of weeks since the chicken pox incident. Bob had just put Henry down for a nap in his room next door. I looked out the window at the gray sky, the bare trees, the dead grass. It was an ugly day. We were having an ugly winter. Everything was cold and brown: no snow, no skiing, no sledding. But it was easier to look at the barren neighborhood than at Bob.

"Renie, I'm fine." He gently touched my knee, trying to bring me back to the room. "I think you're just feeling vulnerable because you're pregnant."

He sounded so calm and sure of what he was telling me, though slightly condescending, as if reassuring a child. He explained that the most common serious ailment for a man his age was a blood cancer, and his bloodwork kept coming back fine.

I wasn't feeling so calm. I sat there calmly enough, staring out the window at the big oak tree in front, resisting his attempts to bring me back into the room, refusing to look at him. If I looked at him, really looked at him, I would be forced to see how he was changing. His skin color was turning gray, his thoughtful blue

17

eyes looked dull and flat, and he carried himself differently and guardedly. He was in pain. He was sick.

≈≈

Bob was my gravity, and without him, I might go spinning off into the stratosphere amidst all the continual planning in my head. Without me, Bob might have spun a web around himself and burrowed in. I kept us connected to people, and he kept us connected to the Earth. It was a pattern developed early on in Oregon.

Bob's journal entry
April 19, 1997

Irene thought we were crazy to leave the cottage for this hike because it was raining and the wind was blowing like crazy. We drove from Cape Cod Cottages to the Cape Perpetua Visitor Center and picked up the trail in the parking lot. The trail was beautiful, lots of old growth. It was all misty and rainy, and the winds would blow hard at times. We saw some big, big trees. Big Dougs and big Spruce. Irene's jacket kept her dry, but the rain doesn't bead up on it anymore like it does on my nice new one. She kept her hood on practically the whole time, even when I told her it wasn't raining anymore. It didn't rain on us too bad during the hike. Afterwards, it really started to pour, though. I love my new boots.

≈≈

When we were living in Portland and would go hiking, I was the one studying the map at the fork in the trail. With my wavy hair sticking out from under my brimmed hat that I purchased at a Grateful Dead concert years before, I'd linger and map-read. I needed to know where we were going and how long it would take to get there and if we had enough food for the trip.

Meanwhile, Bob would be gazing with awe and wonder at the banana slug inching its way across the trail, searching for a log or leaf. A colorful hat from the Portland Saturday Market covered his own shaggy locks. He'd have no worries about the dwindling light or the lack of food.

The air was cool and damp in the forest, and it smelled like the kind of rich soil that has big, fat worms in it. The air we breathed seemed new, untouched by pollutants, filtered by the enormous trees and stirred by the nearby ocean breeze. Looking into the forest from the trail, you could imagine dinosaurs slowly tromping their way through the hillside and casually taking a bite of a nice, big, green, spiky fern.

"Bob, it's getting dusky. We need to get going if we want to get back to the trail head before dark," I would say, a slight edge to my voice.

"Hey, Renie, did you see this Douglas fir? Look at this old growth tree—the sword fern growing out of it wouldn't fit in our kitchen. Amazing," he would muse, as if there were nothing else to focus on at the moment but this tree.

Glancing up from the map, I would see Bob leaning up against the tree with his arms stretched out, as if trying to give the tree a big hug. His arms didn't even make it halfway around the trunk. Those huge old growth trees were an amazing sight.

Thank goodness I had Bob to remind me to pay attention, stop fretting, and enjoy the moment.

Together we had the forest and the trees.

≈≈

We needed both kinds of focus now. We needed one person to pay attention to the details and another to concentrate on the big picture.

I was overwhelmed with symptoms and possibilities, and I needed Bob to keep me grounded in facts. I hadn't told Bob about a conversation I had with our friend, Mike, from Portland. Mike was a new oncology nurse. Mike, his wife, Lori, and their daughter, Raina, had recently visited.

Mike and Lori had been two of our best friends in Portland. They were two of a sixsome, all transplants from Wisconsin who had arrived in the Northwest around the same time. Mark and Amy rounded out the group. Mark and I knew each other from graduate school in Milwaukee. Bob and I came right to their doorstep upon our arrival in town.

The six of us were an interesting bunch. All of us were pale because of our heredity and getting paler from the gray skies of Oregon. Mike was a thoughtful, reserved conversationalist, similar to Bob. Mike had a thin, oval face and the lean limbs of a runner. Mark, who was a runner, was louder about his opinions, with a more agitated kind of energy and hair like Albert Einstein's. Amy often commented that Mark and I must have been related in another life, so similar were our thought processes.

Their wives, Lori and Amy, were both nurses and consistently kind; they had no sarcastic edge like mine. Amy seemed frail when one first met her, but she was as steady and strong as an ox, often finishing up the dishes while the others talked. Rheumatoid arthritis gave Lori a slight limp, but I never heard her complain; her glass seemed half full. I often complained to Bob after a weekend away with the group or a meeting of our short-lived dinner club.

"I think I insulted those two in at least a dozen different ways tonight! I need to find some friends with an edge to them!"

Nonetheless, we spent many weekends away together in tiny cottages on the beach and lodges in the mountains. We all spent leisurely afternoons at Powell's Books. None of us had children yet, and we enjoyed ourselves as young couples with no children could.

Mike had called me a few weeks after their recent visit to Milwaukee to wish me a happy birthday and ask about Bob. He and Lori were worried that his eyes had "lost their spark". I immediately launched into our tale of woe and the litany of Bob's health problems.

Mike's unchecked response: "Weird. That's sometimes how a lymphoma will present itself."

As if tethered to a brick, my heart dropped to my stomach. There was that feeling again, the same one I'd had when I saw Bob leaning over Henry in the bed last fall.

"Remember this moment." I felt more than heard the whispering again.

"You know he's right," this voice told me. My fear continued to whirl around my center, pulling me off balance as I wavered there in the kitchen, clutching the phone.

Then the voice was gone.

Now, days later, as we sat in our guest room, I knew I needed a plan. I needed to take action, but I was scared. I knew there would be no turning back once the plan was in motion. Bob was taking his usual wait-and-see approach. He had more tolerance for the absurdity of a situation; he was more process-oriented.

A few days after the scene in the guest room, I came up the stairs and stopped short on the landing as the floor creaked underneath my weight. I needed no premonition this time; the proof was right there in front of me. Bob was standing in the bathroom, his shirt off, staring into the mirror. He was comparing shoulders, and I could see that one shoulder was bigger than the other, much bigger. *What the hell is going on? What kind of sore muscle is this? I am a trained massage therapist, and this is like no sore muscle I have ever seen. Why is nothing being done about this?*

≈≈

We made another trip to the doctor's office, and finally a CT scan was scheduled.

Bob stood in the kitchen and placed the empty bottle of the white, chalky stuff he had to drink on the counter. The mask of stoicism he had been wearing suddenly became too small to contain the fear behind it, bursting apart. Tears streamed out. Quietly staring, helpless, I stood before him. What could I say? If the situation were reversed, what would Bob say to me? Bob was the rock; I was the dramatic one. If Bob crumbled, I would be groundless, without my gravity.

Bob's desire for honesty and openness with his family came pouring out. He had spent the better part of the winter downplaying or hiding his health issues from his family, but now he thought he was going to need us. He was finally admitting that he was worried and scared. Something might really be wrong.

Bob backed out of the narrow driveway, driving toward the CT scan, toward his destiny. My hand was already on the phone to call my friend Sarah. Sarah and her husband, Garrett, had also met at the bakery. We all had worked there together, and she and I had bonded quickly while bagging the round loaves of bread. We had the same birthday and loved to distract ourselves from our work with conversation; we were soul sisters. Customers would ask frequently if we were actual sisters, and Sarah, with her red hair, would have fit in among my redheaded siblings better than I did, being a sandy blonde.

The dread in my gut was rising at an alarming rate, threatening to block my breathing as I asked Sarah if she could come over and wait with me while Bob got his scan. Remaining composed while Bob fell apart in the kitchen had taxed me. Now that I was on my own, with Henry sleeping upstairs, my cool exterior dissolved.

When Sarah arrived, she was waving a list given to her by Garrett, a new physical therapist. It was a list of conditions that *weren't* cancer and could have caused Bob's health problems. The two of us sat cross-legged on the couch, heads bent over the list. The phone rang. I stared at it as if it were an intruder. When I reluctantly picked it up, Bob was on the other end. His voice was strained and distant as he explained he had been instructed to go directly to the hospital from the CT scan.

Ready or not, here we went.

≈≈

Bob's journal entry
March 28, 2003

Maybe I'm just reluctant to write about this. I was diagnosed with B-cell lymphoma on March 19th.

A doctor who I'd never met before gave me the news.

Okay, I feel like it would take forever to write down everything that has happened in the last two weeks. I do want to process this stuff, but I don't know where to start. Everything is so different today than it was two Saturdays ago. Friday morning was when things really started to fall apart. I went to see an orthopedic doctor about the soreness in my shoulders. He took one look at my shoulder and the cysts on my back and arm and became very concerned. This was where I first really felt fear. This doctor's name was S., and he ordered a CT scan, which he was able to schedule that afternoon. I went from this doctor to another appointment with a surgeon, Dr. M., who concurred with S. in that we were looking at something that was not good. He scheduled me for a biopsy of one of the cysts to be done on Monday in the afternoon. I went home crying. Irene was home, and I told her I was scared, and I cried. I said all sorts of stuff that didn't make any sense, but I think I was just trying to say that I wanted to be honest and open with myself and everyone around me about what I was going through. My family has a tendency to take the go-it-alone approach when it comes to difficult situations, and I wanted to not do this.

I went for the CT scan, and things went from bad to worse. My doctor called me at the imaging center and told me to admit myself to the hospital that afternoon. I called Irene and told her and said I would call again once I was admitted. I was thinking about dying at this point. I remember looking out the window in the imaging center. It was a beautiful day out, and there were birds in a bird feeder right by the window, and I thought about how much I would miss these kinds of experiences. I thought about Henry, and it broke my heart to imagine him without a father. I thought about everything I would miss as he grew up. I thought about Irene and how much I wanted to be with her and how we might not grow old together as I always imagined we would. I thought about dying, and I didn't want to die slow and in pain.

I got to the hospital and I walked up to my room, 3116B. They weren't quite ready for me, which was understandable since things were happening pretty quick. I called Irene and gave her my room number. The nurse brought me a gown and the little padded socks, and all of a sudden I was a hospital patient.

I don't remember who I saw next other then nurses. I think Dr. D. stopped in before Irene arrived. We talked about the CT results and why he admitted me. He said he wanted to treat this thing very aggressively and didn't want to wait until Monday for biopsy results. He had scheduled an MRI that night and had already called an oncologist. At this point he was saying cancer was a possibility, but nothing was for sure. He had also called Irene and told her what was going on. Then Irene arrived.

March 30, 2003

Irene had called my sister Kathy, and Kathy had come over to pick up Henry so Irene could go to the hospital. I know why being married can be such a health benefit because having Irene there was a comfort that couldn't be matched. Anyway, she got there, and I think we kind of girded ourselves for what we imagined we were going to go through. Irene asked if I wanted her to stay the night, and I did. At one point Dr. D. came in and told us about the CT results. We still didn't know anything other than that there was some kind of mass on my kidney and pancreas. Irene left to get some overnight stuff. I was scheduled for an MRI at 8 PM. I was taking Percocet at this point for the tooth and shoulder pain. The CT scan had been pretty painful because I had to lie on my back without moving, and I wasn't really looking forward to doing this again for the MRI. I went down for the MRI, and I told the technicians about the pain in my shoulder. They said I would be in the tube for forty-five minutes and that I should just see how long I could go. They put me on the bench and slid me in. I didn't last two minutes, and my shoulder started throbbing. I was waving my foot and calling out, and they came back in and slid me out. They seemed sympathetic, but they needed to get this done. One of the techs tried putting a pillow under my shoulder, and the other one called up to my nurse's station to see about getting some more Percocet. I went back in the tube to see if the pillow would help, but it didn't and they had to pull me out again. Then they got a hold of Dr. D, and he prescribed a shot of morphine, which did the trick, and we got the MRI done.

When I got back up to my room, Kathy and Jeanne and Irene were there. I told them about the MRI, and we all sat around and talked for a while.

Irene and I watched some television, and then we went to bed.

In the middle of the night an intern came in and woke us up to ask me a bunch of questions that I had already answered.

Saturday Sarah and Garrett came by with Simma's Bakery and Anodyne coffee. They hung out all day long with us. They were there when the doctor told us it was cancer, and it might be a sarcoma. They went AWOL with us to the lakefront. My family met us there, and we gave them the news about me and about Irene, the pregnancy. It was a beautiful day, weatherwise. We all walked for a while on the trail.

We both needed to go AWOL from the hospital that day. We were thinking about self-preservation only. I needed to run like a criminal after a jail break, away from the hospital staff and their forced pleasantries and concerned eyes and their constant questions and probing.

Bob was out of his hospital gown and into the clothes he had worn to the CT scan quicker than you could say "insurance liability". To the inquiring looks from the hospital staff, we simply said that we would be back for Bob's next pain pill.

≈≈

"Is everything OK?" It was my mom on the phone, at long last. I had been trying to reach my mom and dad, who lived in Colorado, ever since Bob went into the hospital the day before. I had been calling all my siblings and trying to locate my parents, but not telling anyone why I so desperately needed to talk to them. Sometimes a month would go by without us talking. My mom knew something had to be very not OK for me to be hunting her down in this way.

I was pacing around and kicking at the dead grass, crushed from the winter cold, Sarah's cell phone pressed to my ear. The four of us, Garret, Sarah, Bob, and I had fled from the hospital and ended up at the park where Bob and I had gotten married just six years earlier. Lake Michigan had looked so blue that day, reflecting the clear sky, and the boats in the marina had looked so inviting. This bleak early spring day was not having the same effect. The lake looked gray and menacing; the air smelled like dead fish.

"No," I choked into the phone, "Bob has cancer."

"Oh, my God," she said in a rush. "What's happening?"

"We don't know. He has a tumor on his kidney and one on his pancreas. His pancreas. His pancreas, Mom. People die of pancreatic cancer." I was choking into the phone.

"I know," she responded slowly, thoughtfully.

"It's all messed up. And there's something else. I'm pregnant," I blurted out.

"Oh, dear," she said evenly.

My mom is half Italian and half British. I think that her calm demeanor and practical approach to living reflect her British heritage. My dad always said that he could come home and tell her he had just been fired or that he had just gotten a large raise and that she and their seven children would have to move fifteen hundred miles away, and her response would be the same: "That's nice, dear. Dinner will be ready in ten minutes."

News of another grandchild should be good news. A cancer diagnosis—this is bad news. Where does a mother go with this information? How does one handle the two opposite extremes of emotion?

"Your dad will come out tomorrow," she stated quietly. It was tax season, after all, and my mom, a tax preparer, was busy with her clients. Sending my dad immediately was the practical tactic.

Thank God! My daddy was going to come out and take care of me. He would bring with him his take-charge attitude, his Irish luck, and his rose-colored glasses. Everything was going to be all right; Dave McGoldrick was coming.

Bob's sisters and mom arrived at the park shortly after my mom and I hung up. They had brought Henry to see us. I wanted to tell them I was pregnant, but Bob was reluctant to share the baby news at this point, thinking the news would be better received once we knew what was going on with his health. He wanted to gather more facts.

Feeling a bit on the theatrical side when it came to Bob's family, I wanted an excuse if I appeared to be falling apart here at the park. The Wellensteins are a Germanic lot, short and sturdy in stature, and they keep most of their emotions to themselves. I usually enjoyed combining my Irish and Italian heritage and spinning a tale with pizzazz, but this time my words were just not coming.

We walked by the lake with everyone. Henry played in the muddy sand puddles left from the melted snow, and all I could think about was raising two kids on my own. Bob's sister, Jane, the more outspoken of the two, and I walked next to each other, and I carried on about Bob's health and my concerns.

"He'll be OK. We just have to figure out what's going on. He's run down," she said, her tone urging me toward optimism.

Wasn't it just a few weeks ago, when I had told her about Bob needing some teeth pulled, that she had expressed concern?

"I'm worried," she had told me then. "Something's going on with his body."

Where was that concern now? I was not just being dramatic; his prospects were not looking good.

During our entire time at the park, Sarah had been nudging me, urging me to tell people I was pregnant, to spit it out. Bob finally told them as we were loading the cars to return home and the hospital.

"Oh, and there's one more thing. Irene's pregnant," he said nonchalantly.

"What?" His mom, Gert, asked as she struggled with her bad knees to get in the car.

Jane was helping her mom swing her legs into the car. "Irene is pregnant," yelled Jane into Gert's better ear.

"Oh, then I'll pray twice as hard," Gert stated. Then she situated herself in the car and looked straight ahead through her thick glasses.

The six of us, Sarah, Garrett, myself, Bob, Kathy and Jane, were trying to get ourselves into the car when this announcement came. Skittishly looking back and forth at each other, we did not know how to react or respond to any of this confluence of information. There were a couple of stiff hugs and quick congratulations and some forced smiles. I felt reluctant to get in the car and drive away from our little oasis.

A minute later, in the back of Sarah and Garrett's old Mercedes, I leaned my head back against the cold leather seat and closed my eyes. I tried to visualize a better scenario for the announcement of the baby. I remembered the thrill around the dinner table when we told Bob's family about Henry. I wanted that electricity, that delight. This baby was supposed to be good news.

"It's not the greatest of timing," as my father said. That was an understatement.

Being pregnant should not be cause for greater concern. The news should not be shrouded in apprehension. But for me, first and foremost, it was. I didn't want to be pregnant right now. I didn't have time for the inconvenience and the worry. How would I raise two kids on my own? I was struggling enough with one, and that was with Bob to help. I could not fathom how I would manage parenthood alone.

The car stopped, and I opened my eyes. We were at the front entrance to the hospital. Its bright lights and the glare on the tiled floor had already become familiar. We obediently followed the color-coded arrows on the tiles to Bob's room, feeling the sting of bleach in our noses. We were resigned. Bob needed more pain medication.

≈≈

The next day my father arrived, and we went directly to the hospital from the airport. Bob's older brother, Eugene, had come to town, and the two men were visiting outside in the courtyard when we arrived. They were ten years apart in age and couldn't have been more different. Bob took after their dad's side of the family in looks, with a more angular face and trimmer build. They both had their dad's industriousness, but Bob had never been as responsible as Eugene, a typical pattern for the youngest and oldest of the family.

As my father and I approached the picnic table, my breath tightened. Next to robust Eugene, Bob looked like a hunched old man. Seeing Bob through my dad's eyes, I couldn't deny how sick he really looked. I had to take note of the dark circles under his eyes and the sallow tone of his skin. I had to control an urge to run up to Bob and stand in front of him, protect him somehow, keep my dad from seeing him in this condition.

≈≈

The oncologist breezed into the room. Dr. Brenda Pierce was a stout young Irish woman with a round, trustworthy, freckled face and a blunt auburn haircut. Businesslike in her neutral colored pantsuit, she looked at the data, and we went chronologically through the same story that we had told countless others in the forty-eight hours since Bob had been admitted.

Had it really only been that long?

Once I finally mentioned the cysts, she started talking about lymphoma. Dr. Pierce was the second medical professional to put our scenario all together. Our friend, Mike, in Portland, had been the first. Mike had diagnosed Bob back in mid-February, from two thousand miles away.

We had been following up on Bob's health concerns from the beginning, when the initial pain in his shoulder had started last fall. But no single doctor whom Bob had seen over those few months had been able to arrive at a diagnosis. He had seen his family doctor, the doctor at the ER, the dentist, and the oral surgeon. Bloodwork had been done and X-rays had been taken, but no one had thought to mention a biopsy of the cysts, even after several had sprung up.

Sitting on the bed with Bob in his hospital room that day, one hand to my stomach and the rapidly dividing cells underneath, I kept asking the oncologist questions. "What if …?"

She kept repeating, in her high staccato voice, that they would do all they could … we would go out of state if we had to. She knew we had a small son to raise. (She only knew half of our situation.)

She put off my questions, repeating the party line: "There's no point in getting ahead of ourselves." She sounded almost cheerful, but distracted, as if her mind had already gone to lab results and treatment plans. And then she breezed back out.

Bob was in a flimsy hospital gown. He looked ridiculous and meek with his knees exposed. Of course the doctor thought he was sick. He looked like a sick person. She should have seen him down at the park earlier, while he was in his clothes.

Weren't we just at home in our cozy living room and lying on the couch under an afghan? Why were we not there, talking about having four stockings hanging above the fireplace next Christmas instead of three?

That doctor obviously didn't know about our plan.

Get her back in here and tell her our plan.

Where did she go now? What was her next step? Could we stop her? Take back Bob's chart? Just forget the whole thing?

We sat on that hospital bed, blood pressure cuffs and IV poles around us. People scurried around just outside the door. At any minute one of those scurrying people could barge in unannounced and poke or prod Bob with something or tell us something else we didn't want to hear.

We sat there like that for a time, like kids who had been scolded and handed a punishment far too harsh for their infraction. Our legs dangled off the sides of the hospital bed. I absently kicked at the mud and dead grass left on my shoes from our excursion to the park; Bob was back in his hospital slippers.

Bob's sister, Kathy, and my dad were waiting somewhere down the hall—a silver-haired, distinguished gentleman in dungarees and a middle-aged woman in jeans and an oversized sweatshirt, turned toward each other in idle conversation, talking about anything but the situation at hand. My dad could carry on a conversation with a stump, and Kathy would add her reflections. They had to have seen the doctor leave, and they must be trying to continue with their small talk, pretending the elephant was not in the hallway with them, waiting for me to come out and tell them what was going on.

What could I tell them? What WAS going on?

Henry was at his Aunt Jane's. Thank goodness, Bob's sisters, Jane and Kathy, had been like second parents to Henry since the beginning, even purchasing a car seat and a portable crib for their place for when they had him overnight. The two of them lived in a duplex together. Jane lived in the upper apartment, and Kathy had the lower. Neither of them had children of their own, and both were perfect aunts.

Kathy had the composure of the seasoned music teacher she was, and Jane was as lively as Kathy was reserved. Kathy was the aunt who sewed fabulous fleece outfits for the boys, her glasses perched on her nose as she concentrated on the needle and thread. Jane was the aunt who riled the kids up with tickling and teasing and then left and let the parents deal with the energy she had created.

What must Henry be thinking now? He was such a thinker. So stoic, Henry could seem like an adult trapped in a child's body. I was so lucky that I did not have to worry about where Henry had been all weekend. I knew he was safe and comfortable with "the aunts".

Bob and I remained motionless, lost in our own thoughts, trying to absorb all that had just occurred.

"So, we're hoping for lymphoma?" I eventually asked Bob. I had sifted the information that the oncologist had just given us and determined that lymphoma was the least offensive option. As unbelievable as that sounds, I was hoping for lymphoma.

"Well, we're hoping it's benign," Bob said slowly.

I inhaled quickly, attempting to dislodge my heart from where it had jumped. It was somewhere in the region of my throat. I looked at Bob sharply.

He can't be serious. This has to be one of his subtle attempts at humor.

I looked for his sly grin, the minuscule head bob, the sidelong glance.

I saw nothing. He wasn't joking. Bob looked back at me, his face as impassive as always. It wasn't going to work this time. He was not going to keep me grounded. He was not able to see how ill he really looked, but I could. The realist in me told me "benign" was not even a remote option.

I immediately jumped into my planner role: *What happens next? What do we do now? Where will we be when … ? What do we have to do to get there?*

Bob jumped into his scientific observer role: *Let's gather all the facts, get all the information, think about it, and remain calm. It will all be figured out in due time.*

There and then began our separate journeys. These two journeys were both part of the same story, but there would be different endings for the two of us. We found ourselves at another fork in the road. This time, however, we were taking different paths. But we complemented each other still, picking up each other's slack to proceed with the task at hand and get the job done.

≈≈

"My husband has lymphoma!" I wanted to shout from the rooftops. I was so elated. Lymphoma was the least of all the possible evils; it was the diagnosis I had hoped for.

Bob had just told me the news as we walked back home from dropping Henry off at day care. The early spring air felt cool and moist and smelled like earth freshly turned.

"Wait, when did you find out? How long have you known?" I inquired, suddenly suspicious.

"Yesterday."

"You knew this yesterday?" I couldn't believe it.

"I didn't want to ruin your massage last night," he responded.

Lymphoma had not been the news Bob hoped for. It wasn't good news for him. Trying to make sense of the information himself, he had been trying to spare me the bad news. Bob had still entertained "benign" as an option. It had still been an option for him until the tests came back with a definitive answer.

Now there was no more speculation, no more possibilities. He stood, stranded on the street, facing me. He was reluctant to admit the truth. He wasn't ready to redefine himself. He wanted to reject the label.

"I have lymphoma," he slowly repeated the statement. As he looked me straight in the eyes, I could hear our breathing come more rapidly.

We stood there on the sidewalk with the word "lymphoma" bobbing and dipping around us. It eventually settled down beside us. I saw him pick it up and step into the word. He pulled it up around him and zipped it up like a snowsuit.

My husband had cancer.

≈≈

Our plan now involved eight sessions of chemo, remission, a possible stem cell transplant, and a baby. We had it very organized and conveniently planned.

Wrapped in an afghan, I curled in the fetal position on the couch in the living room. It was Bob's first weeks of chemo, and I felt sick, early-pregnancy sick. Bob should be making me tea and the perfect meal, preferably something comforting that my mom would have made. Couldn't he read my mind? Didn't he remember I was pregnant?

"And there it goes," Bob sang out.

Seated at the dining room table, he was correcting papers and literally tearing his hair out. I could see the strands in his hands from where I lay. His hair fell out faster than either of us imagined it would.

Silently I cursed our circumstances.

I couldn't ask him to make me tea. I couldn't "pull a roommate", as we often said to each other. This phrase was coined in college by my housemates, and we used it when one person was too lazy to do something and would ask the other person to do it since that person was up.

The man had cancer; I should be taking care of him. What about the fact that I was creating life? He was supposed to be fawning over me and worrying about me, not the other way around. *Pregnancy doesn't trump cancer*, I concluded, feeling sorry for myself.

It was all about Bob now. I got up to start the water for tea.

≈≈

Later that week, Bob and I sat across from each other at our oval dining room table amidst books on lymphoma. We had just returned from the baby's first ultrasound, and Bob had lumbered in with all these books from the library. I couldn't help thinking of Henry's first ultrasound. We had hurried to the library afterwards to get a book about fetal growth and development.

My dad had gone home earlier that day, before the ultrasound. I had watched his rented car drive away from our house and toward the airport from the window in our second floor guest room. I had to stifle my intense urge to run after him. I envisioned myself running after the car and waving him down—"Don't leave me, Daddy, please don't leave me here all alone. Please." But he left with visions of Bob's miraculous recovery in his head.

And now here I sat, eight weeks pregnant, a two-and-a-half-year-old running around the house and doing God knows what—he was in a throwing phase at the time. Bob and I were busy reading through the stacks of information. I was reading statistics comparing lymphoma to non-Hodgkin's lymphoma.

"I am sure glad you don't have non-Hodgkin's," I casually said to Bob, not even looking up from the book.

"Why?" he responded, his interest piqued.

"Because the statistics aren't nearly as good for non-Hodgkin's," I said. My eyes remained on the page.

"Renie, I do have non-Hodgkin's." Bob spoke quietly but firmly.

"No, you don't," I responded sharply. I finally looked up from the book. I was surprised by his stern tone.

"Yes, I do." Now he was almost chuckling, as if we were playing.

"No, you don't," I countered, not playing.

"Why do you think the doctor gave me all these brochures about non-Hodgkin's lymphoma, then?" He waved his hand across the table, gestured toward the brochures and her neatly written notes, presenting me with the proof. "Renie, I have non-Hodgkin's lymphoma." Bob was calm again, as if he were explaining to Henry why he shouldn't touch a hot stove.

My eyes darted towards the brochures and back to the book with the evil statistics, then back to Bob.

"No, you don't," I pleaded, pounding my fist on the book. "No, you don't."

Bob's journal entry
March 16, 2003

Dear Henry,

I don't know how to begin to tell you how much I love you.

You are 2 ½ years old and I so enjoy being a part of your life. I hope I am going to be a part of it for a long, long time.

You are a wonderful child. You are filled with love and energy and curiosity. I love coming home to hear what you have to say and to hear about all of your adventures. I love to hug you and read books to you and walk around the block with you. I love to build towers with you and play with your trains and your play dough that you and your mom make.

I want you to explore both yourself and this incredible world we live in. You and I live in this world together.

That cannot be changed, Henry.

At one point you and I lived together in the world.

Chapter Two

Rock Bottom

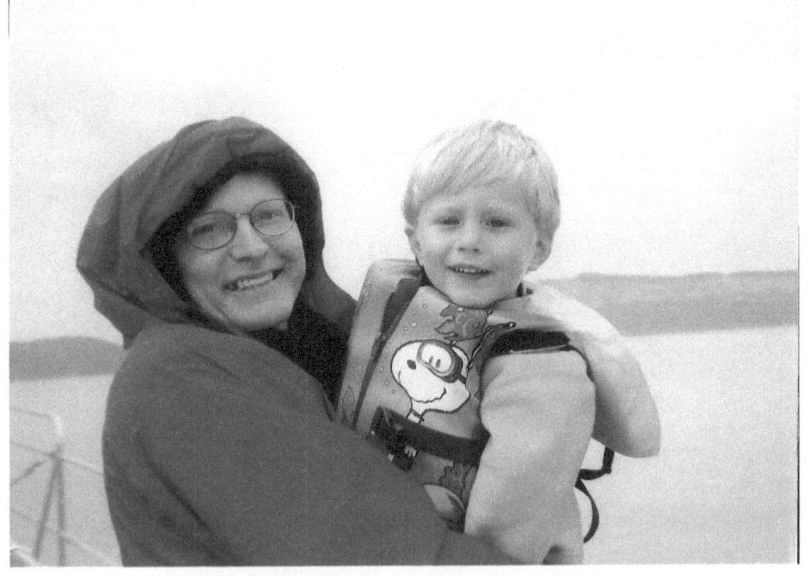

Life is a succession of readjustments.
Elizabeth Bowen

"Are we going to radiation today, Daddy?" Henry asked Bob above the roar of the blender. Bob was fixing Henry's morning smoothie.

It was July, and Bob was done with work for the summer. He was now going for a radiation treatment to his shoulder every weekday. Forty-five radiation treatments were part of his preparation for a stem cell transplant in Nebraska.

Bob's treatment was not going according to plan. The stem cell transplant was the new plan, and it wasn't the first revision to the original plan. We were four months into this cancer journey, and I was tired.

We had about three, maybe six, good weeks following his initial diagnosis on March 21, 2003. All the tumors went away. Bob was pain-free, and his energy was better than it had been in months. He had a little spring in his step again, which I found nothing short of miraculous.

"I feel like we've gotten off easy," Bob said one night as we were turning out the lights.

"Shhhhh, don't say that, you will tempt the fates," I replied quickly, shuddering as I heard the secret speak to me again.

"*Not so quickly,*" was its chilling whisper.

I was tired of disappointing news from the doctor. The continual questions and the need to keep track of so many appointments wore on me. About the only major concern I wasn't tired of was my pregnancy. As long as I was pregnant, it meant I still only had one child to worry about; the baby was the safest one among us.

I was tired of worrying.

Henry and Bob's chatter made its way up the stairs as I stood at the blue sink in the bathroom off the landing, getting ready for work. I paused to look at myself in the mirror. Did I look like I was OK? Did I look like myself? How must I look to others? I looked normal, right? I looked like Irene, a functioning human being, a responsible adult, a parent, a spouse, a social worker. Could I pull this act off today at work? Could I actually get any work done with all the noise in my head? Could I stand all the concern and the questions today from all of our well-meaning friends and family?

It was exhausting to have so many people caring about us.

My hand reflexively went to my chest. Could people see my heart, glaring and harsh, dangling like an exposed light bulb switched on in a dark basement? It didn't feel warm and inviting. A person's first impulse would be to shut his eyes or turn away from the intrusive brightness.

The energy of my anxiety buzzed around me. I hoped I wouldn't explode as light bulbs sometimes do when they burn out. People near me would hear a quick pop, followed by that tinkling sound as I hit the floor.

I desperately wanted to maintain some kind of control.

"Renie, do you want some chai?" Bob called up the stairs, bringing me back to the present moment.

"RENIE, DO YOU WANT SOME CHAI?" mimicked Henry, followed by the familiar *skrrrrr* of the espresso machine Bob used to froth my chai every morning, the warm smell of cinnamon floating up the stairs.

Henry loved going to radiation with Bob that summer. What's not to love about radiation? The girls there were so nice to him, and he got to see Daddy on the TV screen. The radiology technicians let him stay with them and watch the TV, set up behind a big glass window, instead of remaining out in the waiting area. Henry intently and quietly absorbed all the procedures Bob had to go through.

Henry was blissfully unaware that the radiation was a desperate attempt to remove the cancer from his dad's body just long enough to hit him with high-dose chemo and replenish his system with fresh stem cells, giving his body a fresh start. All Henry knew was that he got to choose a treat after Bob was done with his treatment, and that was cool.

I, on the other hand, was not enjoying my summer activities nearly as much as Henry was enjoying his. Five months pregnant at that point, I needed to get the show on the road so I didn't deliver a baby while still in Nebraska.

I needed the radiation to shrink the tumor, Bob's blood levels to remain stable, and the body scan (PET scan) following the treatments to be clear of any cancer activity. And I needed all this to be done so we could get to Omaha, Nebraska, and start the seven-week stem cell transplant procedure by early September.

I had to fill out forms so I could take family leave from work, find an ob-gyn doctor in Omaha, figure out what would happen with Henry while Bob and I were in the hospital, figure out what would happen when we were all outpatients, and much more.

You would think I would have loved it—all that planning.

Remaining there, rooted to the worn tiled floor, I stared at myself in the bathroom mirror. Unbidden, lists formed in my head. I flashed abruptly back to July 7, three weeks earlier, when we had hit rock bottom. Or so I had thought. It seemed that we had been at rock bottom several times now. Little did I know how far we still had to go before we actually got to rock bottom.

≈≈

Our first arrival at rock bottom was in May, when Bob neglected to tell me the tumor in his shoulder had come back. The right shoulder, just to the left of the scapula and the right of the spine, was where Bob had first started to complain about pain back in the fall. It was the original site. Bob began to feel something there again in between the second and third rounds of chemo, but he remained silent on the subject.

When I innocently answered the phone one evening and heard Bob's oncologist start telling me the results from Bob's latest round of tests, I fully expected to hear he was in remission. I had no reason to believe otherwise.

Reluctantly she told me there was still a "hot spot" in the shoulder, meaning that there was still cancer activity in his body.

"Everything else looked great," she stated. "There was nothing on the kidney, nothing on the liver or pancreas anymore. He is only through three rounds, remember. There is still plenty of time," she continued.

My heartbeat began revving up. *Why wasn't she saying the word? Why was she not saying 'remission'?*

"Now, what about the tumor on his shoulder? Does Bob think that's any worse?" she haltingly asked, unaware of the eruption she was about to cause.

"I don't know anything about the tumor on his shoulder," I curtly replied as I lost control of my heart, which went slipping down in my chest. Caught off guard, I froze momentarily, suddenly panicked. Kicking into fight or flight mode, I began to pace around the house, my mind racing in another direction, away from the conversation on the phone.

Had Bob been acting differently, melancholy maybe?

"Have Bob call the office to schedule an appointment," I heard the doctor say somewhere in the din. Placing the phone down, I steadied myself with the counter, attempting to take a deep breath and calm my speeding heart. Ignoring my efforts, it kept its wild pace while my mind wandered, unleashed, into the past two weeks.

Bob had seemed weary and depressed, that I knew, but I thought the third round of chemo had just started to catch up with him. He was perplexed and brooding about this experiment in which he was the subject. Bob enjoyed the research aspect of this dilemma; the challenge appealed to him. All the new jargon he was learning and the fascinating procedures and drug concoctions and interactions with his body were alluring in an objective way. But the solution was not coming easily. Every time he thought he had found his way out of the maze, thus far, he had actually reached another dead end.

Bob was bewildered by his lack of success with this little science experiment.

I began to see how Bob's omission had manifested itself in subtle but insidious ways in our daily lives. He had become more introspective and less talkative; without realizing how I was responding, I had become more hyper and controlling to compensate.

Being Bob, he continued to go about his daily routines of cooking, going to work, making lesson plans, biking, hanging out with Henry, and doing all his chores around the house. He masked any uncertainty with dogged determination to keep up with his responsibilities.

The significance of the early recurrence of the cancer on Bob's physical well-being was lost on me amongst my greater concern for our emotional well-being. If he didn't tell me about the tumor on his shoulder coming back, what else was he not telling me? What was going on in that head of his? What was he thinking?

My life had become an open book. All I did was talk, fret, plan, and emote. I talked to my coworkers, my family, Bob's family, health care professionals, friends, Bob, Henry, more family members, and yet more friends.

Who was Bob talking to? Our conversations were very task-oriented these days, I suddenly realized: *What did we need to do, when should we do it, how were we going to get there, who would watch Henry, did so-and-so call back, did you read this article?*

Bob never used two words if he could get away with one, a trait I had always admired, since I am so detail-oriented. But this silence was intolerable in our high-stakes situation.

Following the fateful phone call with the oncologist, I had to leave right away to give a massage. The next morning at 6:00 AM, I was leaving for my brother Mike's wedding in Colorado. Now I had to talk to Bob about his medical situation, one more wrench in my planning.

Bob came home from work that evening to these scribbled, cryptic notes I had taken while talking to the doctor. How would he know that "(-) liver" meant that there was nothing on the liver? He thought the opposite: negative liver, *bad liver, liver bad*. Bob had arrived home to Henry, his sister, Jane and Jane's friend, Ann, and these scribbles, thoughtlessly left on the island in the kitchen.

When I returned home following the massage, we had the worst argument of our relationship. Leaning against opposite counters in our kitchen, the spicy smell of ginger from dinner still lingering around us, we faced each other as if we were boxers waiting for the bell.

"I didn't want to worry you. I hoped the tests would come back good and you would've never had to know." Aggravatingly level-headed, Bob defended his inaction.

"Why would you want to worry alone? Jeez, Bob, I would tell you if I had a hangnail. What about all that bullshit about needing your friends and family? This is happening to me too, Bob, but I have no control over the information I get. You can't go it alone this time. Not this time." I gestured wildly for emphasis.

"I'm sorry, Renie. I will tell you everything from now on," he promised, sounding remorseful.

"Don't worry! You won't have to tell me anything. I'm going with you to every appointment from now on," I vowed.

In an attempt to proceed with our life, our relationship, and our family, we had been trying to keep our routines as normal as possible "for Henry". We had been telling each other that Bob's cancer was a bump in the road, a storm to weather until our lives got back to normal, a not-so-subtle reminder to appreciate our lives.

It was becoming increasingly obvious that we were not getting out of this illness maze very easily.

Maintaining our standard of independence, coupled with the reality of our young family, meant that Bob had been going to appointments with friends and family or by himself. My dad had gone with Bob to his first session, and our friend, Sarah, had gone with him to subsequent treatments.

The staff at the clinic thought Sarah was Bob's wife. She and I are often mistaken for sisters, and we are very close, but enough was enough. Now that I no longer trusted him to keep me informed, I feared our self-reliance was about to be compromised.

Bob's journal entry
May 3, 2003

All this fear. Fear of something I can't stop. Fear of getting shoved over a cliff. I hate the idea of dying that way but then again I love it. The short trip knowing where you are going mostly. I know I have to die someday but not now. I really don't want to die now.

Yesterday Irene and Henry and I went to the park. It was freezing cold. The sun was out but the wind was blowing in off the lake and Henry was the only one dressed warm enough. He was having a great time while I was constantly looking for something to stand behind to break the wind.

We saw a wood duck. There is a pair of wood ducks that I've seen there before and I was telling Irene about them when the one turned up. I worried that he or she had lost their mate.

As I was looking to get out of the wind behind the band shell I came across a finch flittering around in a bush. What a restless bird, almost like a hummingbird. It covered every square inch of this bush inside and out. I called Henry over and he watched it intently. At one point it flew out of the bush and landed on the path right in front of Henry as if it was checking him out. Henry was surprised and flinched a little but he had a smile on his face. It was great to see that smile.

I'm tired and angry at this cancer. I don't want to do it anymore. I don't want to worry. I don't want to sit in that fucking chemo chair anymore. I don't want to have to go through anymore of these scans. I don't want to see any more doctors or nurses or receptionists.

I love the sympathy though. Sometimes I work it. I act more tired than I am. At school I try to make it obvious how out of breath I am when I walk up the stairs. When people ask me how I am doing I say 'I'm doing all right' in a tone that conveys what I'm really doing is keeping a stiff upper lip. This is all such a joke though because what I'm really hiding is how afraid I am and how much I hate this whole thing. I feel like I'm always in that PET scan tube and I can't move and I can't change what is happening to me and I just have to let all the drugs course into my body.

Journal Entry
May 20, 2003

I'm missing two teeth. I might lose two more. I hate losing teeth. It seems so permanent. It's not like skin flaking off or even hair falling out. Who cares about hair? I can eat without hair. Teeth are like arms or maybe fingers. I'm very appreciative of my teeth now.

My back is causing me some discomfort again. I still have cancer. I thought it was gone but it is not.

I want to live a long, long time but I might not. Everybody can say that. I have cancer though so it's optimistic of me to imagine living for the foreseeable future.

I don't know if I am really taking this seriously. Probably not but why the hell should I. Of course I don't want to die but I have to eventually and I would rather embrace the idea as just another aspect of life than be emotionally paralyzed by the idea of death.

If this turns out bad, I'm going to be afraid and I'm going to be terribly sad. I wanted to spend a long life with Irene. I want to see my children grow up and enjoy life with them. I want to explore more of this world. I want to become more of who I am.

≈≈

Memorial Day weekend marked our second arrival at rock bottom.

Bob was supposed to get a biopsy of the tumor on his shoulder so the doctor could determine if we were still dealing with the same type of lymphoma or if it had morphed into something different.

The morning of the appointment, Bob rode his bike, with Henry in tow, to the park to meet some friends. Willy, a mellow folk musician with a strawberry blonde goatee and a come-as-you-are attitude, whom we had met in birth class, offered some grapes to the group standing around the sandbox. Bob grabbed a couple.

After arriving home, smelling like suntan lotion and sand, Bob suddenly realized that he was supposed to be fasting for the surgery. Knocking his head like a V8 commercial, he casually chastised himself for the mistake.

I could not be so casual about his lapse. "Are you sabotaging your recovery, Bob? What were you thinking?" I yelled at him while marching around the kitchen, flailing my arms.

"I didn't think about it. Willy just handed me some grapes. I took some grapes." Bob explained, shrugging his shoulders, head tilted to one side, arms out in an "oh well" expression. He appeared bemused by my overreaction.

"Now what are we supposed to do?" I screeched, frantic.

It was Friday, and now we had to wait over the entire holiday weekend because you can't get these procedures done on weekends or holidays.

"Cancer doesn't grow on the weekends," as my sister Teri said.

Oh, how I wish that were true. At this point I could literally see the tumor get bigger by the day. It was horrifying. Once the biopsy finally was done, we would have to wait again for the results and then wait again for the doctor to make her determination. Wait, wait, wait—I couldn't wait.

"Just don't tell them." I suggested in a burst of desperation. "Just go—what are they going to do?"

He had just eaten a couple of grapes, and they are mostly water, I reasoned. I wanted Bob to get that offensive growth biopsied now.

I stood in the kitchen, defiant, arms crossed, listening to him on the phone. He mentioned the grapes, he nodded his head, and I heard the word *Tuesday*. Grabbing my purse off the counter, I turned on my heel and headed for the grocery store in a huff.

Finding myself in the diaper aisle, I stood gaping at the prices, a number I hadn't noticed in a while. Henry would be three in July, and we were planning on starting toilet training when we returned from my family's reunion at the end of June. We would be traveling to the San Juan Islands off Washington, and we didn't want a newly trained child on a trip that involved planes, trains, ferries, and automobiles.

Continuing to stare at the rather large number before me, I began to calculate in my head. Soon we would have a second child, and that number could possibly double.

"No way, not going to happen," I thought.

I left the aisle without putting anything in the cart.

"Where's Henry?" I asked Bob when I returned from the store and found him sitting in his La-Z-Boy, journaling, a steaming cup of chamomile tea beside him.

"Napping," he said hesitantly, glancing up from his writing, waiting for my head to either explode or start spinning around.

"OK, here's the deal. When he gets up, we are telling him that there are no more diapers, that the diapers are all gone." I said this with conviction, leaving no room for debate.

"OK," he responded even more hesitantly, picking up his tea and breathing in the fresh calming scent, eyes on me.

"Listen, it's going to be a crappy weekend anyway, so we might as well just deal with crap all weekend," I retorted as I left the room.

Later, after we had broken our news to Henry and he was back to sleep for the night, (it is a wonder he ever went to sleep again—he might well have wondered *what else might disappear while I am sleeping, my car seat?*) Bob and I prepared to watch *The Sopranos*. I was on the couch, listening to the opening song.

In walked Bob with a plate of glistening purple grapes, offering them to me as if they were an olive branch. He was wearing that sheepish smile of his.

I had seen that same sheepish smile on a trip we took to Europe while we were living in Portland. We had spent a week in Ireland with my family for one of our regular reunions and then took off to visit Sarah and Garrett, who were living in Amsterdam at the time.

Bob and I visited Belgium by ourselves and spent a day in the enchanting town of Brugge. Every building and every street provided a picture-taking moment. I was snapping away the entire day.

As we stood on the platform, waiting for our train back to Brussels, I talked nonstop, reliving our storybook day. Bob was intent on the camera, not paying a lick of attention to me. I became suspicious, and he finally admitted that it appeared that he had forgotten to put a new roll of film in the camera. (This was before the days of digital cameras.)

All those pictures I had taken all day long did not exist. Near tears, like a child begging her parents for a ride on a pony, complete with jumping up and down, I grabbed Bob's arm and tried to convince him to go back into town and retrace our steps.

"Ah, Renie, cheer up. We'll always have Brugge," Bob told me, trying to lighten the mood with some corny *Casablanca* quote.

"Look, I think you can allow me a moment to be upset about this. We will never be back here, and now we have no pictures. You know how important pictures are to me." I was miffed by his humor.

My hair blew back as the train arrived. I stormed on, not sparing him a backward glance. The train was crowded, and I took the first seat I saw, leaving Bob to fend for himself. We sat separately for a few stops until the crowd thinned. Even after there was room for us to sit together, I stayed stubbornly where I was. Bob stood up and came over.

"Is this seat taken?" he asked cautiously.

I shrugged, and he sat down. Our arms brushed, and my agitation dissipated. The next morning we were having breakfast at a little café before taking the Chunnel to London. Bob excused himself with little explanation. I sat there, perplexed, looking at my watch. He returned and handed a package to me. In the bag was a calendar for the next year, 1998.

All the pictures in the calendar were of Brugge.

The tangy grapes Bob offered me that night are long gone, of course, but I still have the calendar, reminding me of Bob and the ingenious ways he had of taking care of me, of us, by defusing a tense situation with a small, thoughtful gesture and a casual smile.

≈≈

Bob's journal entry
June 17, 2003

I'm starting round two of the new chemo regimen. I actually started it yesterday but today I begin the 24 hour segment. I have a substitute administering my exams today and tomorrow. I will hopefully be able to make it into school tomorrow afternoon to do the grades and then around 6:00 PM we will leave for Angie's house and then Thursday morning we fly out of O'Hare for the San Juans.

What if I am cured? What if I am given my life back? What will I do differently?

- I will set aside time for meditation and yoga
- I will join a rock climbing gym
- I will get into therapy
- I will pay attention to my emotions
- I will draw and paint

≈≈

Our oncologist thought we were nuts to place so much importance on my family reunion, located in the San Juan Islands near Seattle, Washington. It had been planned for three years. We had to get back to the Northwest, where our relationship had been rooted, where we had been at our best, where the air smelled of the wet salty sea, and everywhere you looked, there was new life.

That trip was as important for our morale as good blood results would have been at that point. We would have gone AWOL again if we had to.

Henry was an amazing traveler, and we had many moments when we were able to convince ourselves that we were just a normal family on vacation, enjoying the great outdoors.

Then, during a whale-watching excursion, I noticed Bob holding onto Henry's bright yellow life jacket on the upper deck of the boat. Henry kept leaning out over the railing, displaying his zest for life at the expense of the adults surrounding him. Watching my two boys from inside the cabin, I noticed a difference in Bob.

His eyelashes are falling out. His brows too—damn, he looks like a cancer patient.

Up until that moment, to me, Bob had looked like a good-looking bald man. Now he looked like a cancer patient, a good-looking cancer patient.

≈≈

"Bob is such a good dad, Irene," said Kathy, number two among my siblings and a bit of a worrier. We were back at the resort, seated on a bench, watching Henry and Bob canoe around the inlet where our cabins looked out at the Pacific Ocean. Bob was most likely pointing out a hawk or eagle to Henry as they bobbed on the water; he seemed determined to pass his fascination with these unsociable birds on to Henry, who already had the watchful part down.

"I know. They have a wonderful symmetry to them." I nodded, not taking my eyes off the two of them. Bob had always been more natural with Henry than I was; he understood him instinctively.

I continued my attempt to store up memories on this trip, like a squirrel gathering nuts for the winter. I wished they could stay out there forever, just the two of them. If I watched them together enough, could I store up enough memories to last a lifetime? Could I figure out Bob's secret for parenting?

Never having a great maternal instinct, I never had a huge desire to have a child. Figuring that Bob could make up for what I lacked, I had great confidence in our ability to raise a family together. I trusted Bob and his cool logical thinking, believing it was the perfect balance to my restless, critical nature.

Selfish and not particularly nurturing, I had a high need for independence and an equally high expectation for personal responsibility from others. Feeling needed anchored me. That is why Bob and I worked as well as we did, even though both of us were so independent.

Our relationship felt decadent and practical at the same time to me. How could I have known that I would meet someone who would wrap around me like a favorite blanket of just the perfect weight and softness? I wanted to curl up on the couch wrapped up in the comfort of Bob.

Bob and I were a great team, maintaining equilibrium together. I wanted to raise children with him. I wanted the two of us to be pregnant together and labor together and parent together.

Just as I might have expected, I did not take to motherhood well initially. Henry was not a contented baby, and I took that fact very personally. He did not cry; he *screamed*, and he did it frequently. He wouldn't nap, and he was never happy to just sit and watch the world go by. Once he could roll over, he screamed until he could crawl, and then he screamed until he could walk—and then he had to run. Henry was a child in constant motion.

I would see other babies in their strollers, bouncy seats, or high chairs, just sitting and looking out at their world. Not Henry, who sat in a bouncy seat for exactly two minutes, climbed out of high chairs, and never tolerated a stroller. The two of us walked around the neighborhood with two strollers. I pushed one while Henry pushed the other. Outdoors and not restricted in any way, Henry was at his happiest.

I tried to tell myself that all these tendencies I found so aggravating were signs of intelligence and that I hadn't made an enormous mistake by becoming a mother. When I was anxious or upset, Henry grew anxious and upset, and I resented having my emotions reflected back at me so blatantly. Resenting Henry's neediness, I terribly missed Bob and the relationship I had with my husband before Henry.

One autumn evening when Henry was about fifteen months old, I took him outside to enjoy the gloaming, my favorite time of day. The sky was turning pink, and the leaves on the trees shimmered red and orange as the chill in the air hit them.

Henry, however, was not interested in the gloaming or its seductive colors. He was too busy ignoring my warnings and running into the street, once, twice, and then a third time. Three times—he was out! I stormed down the driveway and scooped him up, not very gently, convinced he had done this on purpose just to piss me off.

"He ruined it for me! I'd been looking forward to being outside all day," I complained to my therapist at our next meeting.

"Irene, he's fifteen months," she reminded me gently as I recounted this tale to her, still seething, days later. "You don't actually think he did this to make you mad, do you?"

"Yes, I do," I stated, sure of myself. "You don't know him."

"Irene, he's fifteen months. That's what fifteen-month-olds do," she restated.

"I just wanted to enjoy the gloaming, I had looked forward to it all day," I trailed off, realizing how selfish and ridiculous I must sound.

In retrospect, I feel that I was completely unrealistic about a baby's impact on my life. I had imagined that I would give birth to a five-year-old, a being who could reason and share my view of the world. I imagined that I would give him massages, and he would be very serene. I was ignorant of the fact that a child comes into the world with their own temperament and that we parents must help our children best utilize their skills, whatever those abilities are or are not.

I eventually realized that I resented Henry for bringing about the change in the relationship between Bob and me. Having a mom who grew up feeling resented by her mother, I refused to have Henry grow up feeling resentment from me. My therapist helped me to see that Henry's behavior was normal. Time and the leveling out of hormones eventually had me back to myself and feeling more capable. But that process took until Henry was about eighteen months old, and they were eighteen long months.

Bob was able to incorporate Henry into his life more easily and had a more detached, observant style. He didn't take everything so personally. Henry had Bob's way of looking at the world, as if it were one big experiment to figure out, but he also had my impatient nature. It was a tough temperamental combination for a child because experiments take time and patience.

I had no patience with Henry's impatience. To make matters worse, Henry had no patience with his own impatience either. Henry's nature was constantly at odds with itself. On one hand, he was watchful, a kid who needed to get the lay of the land before he would venture into a new situation. On the other hand, he was intolerant and edgy, sensitive to too much stimulation but capable of creating a lot of it all on his own.

Henry would cruise across our wood floors from one side of the living room to the other on his Radio Flier scooter at top speed and crash into the back door—*bang*! He would do this again and again. Thank goodness the door had a kick guard on it.

Lacking the self-confidence required to take his show on the road, Henry became shy and reserved when out of his element, immediately going into his observant mode. My coworkers never believed my stories of his loud antics at home. At my workplace, he never said a word, just looked at people with this intense look that became known as "the Henry Stare", as if he were seeing beyond them or trying to escape within.

An astrologer friend of mine told me Henry was a "triple fire". His sun, moon and rising sign are all fire signs. But he also has lots of water in his chart, more calming and reflective. Having absolutely no air in his chart, it is hard for him to find balance. Easily frustrated by actions or objects that he was not able to master immediately, he would go tense all over, and he would turn red with his attempt to control his irritation. When he couldn't hold it in anymore, he would erupt with a roar.

"There's his triple fire," Kathryn, the astrologer, would say.

Mortified by his behavior, unable to ride out the storm, I would attempt to assist with the task, resulting only in increased agitation.

Henry and I whipped each other up, but Bob and Henry's energies complemented each other in the same way Bob's and mine did.

Bob was the great stabilizer for us all.

Bob's journal entry
July 30, 2000

Henry is a beautiful baby. This past week has been amazing. It's just crazy that Irene and I and this new little guy are all together here. I'm amazed that I have this responsibility of keeping this little guy safe and sound and reasonably content. Irene of course has the lion's share of keeping him content but I do what I can. If he cries before it's time to eat, I walk with him and rock and do whatever I can. I love holding him, even when he cries—and can he ever cry. He has this crying overdrive that makes him sound like a cornered wolverine. It's almost unnatural sounding, coming from this adorable little person.

≈≈

The last night of the San Juan reunion, the entire family was seated at four top tables eating dinner. While the sun set over the Pacific Ocean and the gardens filled with pink and red rhododendrons, the subject of the next reunion came up. According to the McGoldrick custom, the couple hosting the next reunion, three years from the current one, announced the location.

Italy! The excitement traveled around the room from table to table.

I sat frozen in my seat with a stiff smile on my face. Did no one else hear that, feel that? It was the secret. It was back. I felt a cold hand squeeze my heart; the hair on my arms rose.

"*Pay attention,*" it whispered, getting louder. "*You won't be here again, not like this.*"

I glanced nervously around the room. No one seemed to notice the grip that had me stunned. Then it vanished as quickly as it had come, leaving me winded and wondering.

What would my life be like in 2006? Would Bob be with us? If he was, would he be healthy? Would we ever take those Italian classes we had been talking about?

≈≈

Bob and I knew his medical progress was not going well, but we did not understand just how badly. We should have had an inkling when Bob's doctor had cried at the appointment following the first recurrence in the shoulder. At the time I thought she was just an unusually sensitive doctor and that she liked us a lot and was sympathetic to our young family.

Our friend Mike (the oncology nurse) knew how serious the situation was, especially after we noticed that the tumor was coming back a second time, when we arrived in Portland after the reunion. We asked Mike to palpate Bob's shoulder one evening. He remained noncommittal despite our inquisitive faces.

"That's just his muscle there, right, Mike?" I implored. My gaze moved between Mike's face and Bob's shoulder. Knowing the mass was there, small but there, I didn't want to focus on either one of them.

It was reassuring for me to visit Mike and Lori on that trip. Their nursing expertise was a great relief. They helped me flush the peripherally inserted catheter (PIC line) Bob now had in his arm for the continued treatment and reassured me about blood counts.

Bob was determined to not be a sick person while traveling. He started by refusing a wheelchair at the airport even though he had just finished chemo the day before. By the time we were in Portland, he was feeling rather good and wanted to hike and do all the activities we had been yearning for the past three years.

Bob was usually the inspiration and motivation for our outdoor activities when we lived in Portland. This trip was no different. He and Mike took Henry and their daughter, Raina, on a hike to Ape Cave at the South base of Mt. St. Helen's, a hike we had done while living in Portland. It was a hike that Bob had especially enjoyed. We girls opted for a child-free day in the city.

There were the usual mishaps that most adventures with Bob involved. The four spelunkers arrived at a dead end in the cave. Bob had expected a ladder to lead them out of the cave, but no ladder was there, only a narrow shaft towards the ceiling of the cave. Expecting to find the ladder at the end of the shaft, Bob shimmied through the narrowing space while Mike stayed with the kids. Eventually the shaft ended—still no ladder. Bob scooted back out to the place where Mike was entertaining the weary children by turning off the flashlights so they could listen to the drippy darkness of the cave as the stalactites loomed large above their heads.

Bob calmly pondered the possibilities, believing the ladder had to be somewhere. They just had to keep plodding along until they found it. He had no worries about agitated children or flashlights running out of batteries. He eventually did find the ladder. Such calculated risks often turned out well for Bob.

So where was the ladder to lead him out of his cancer? Bob remained calmly confident that the ladder was somewhere; we just hadn't found it yet.

Mike did not provide comfort to Bob as much as he did to me, I am afraid. There was an evening when the two of them went out. Mike wanted to talk to Bob about how he felt about dying and how it affected our relationship.

Bob was insulted by those questions. At that point, he did not understand how dire his prospects were and had no interest in discussing dying and all the implications involved with that. He wanted support and positive thinking. In Mike's defense, Mike understood the implications of the first treatment's swift failure; the second did not appear to be working either. It wasn't easy to meet Bob at that point of his journey. We were all on our own journeys.

Bob's journal entry
July 5, 2003

Tonight, I turned on the TV and nothing was on.
I surfed between *Scream 2* and a *Star Trek* movie

(*First Contact*). I felt the guilt and boredom of sitting mindlessly watching TV. My sisters are having a margarita party tonight. Irene and I were going to make an appearance with Henry but we skipped it. We were both feeling pretty tired and Henry was starting to fall apart but I still feel guilty for not going.

I think we are all three still recovering from our trip to the Northwest.

I'm feeling on the verge of depression. I have some soreness in my back and I worry constantly that the cancer has returned. I went to see "Bowling for Columbine" with Mike H. out in Portland. Afterwards we went to the Barley Mill. Mike asked how my relationship with Irene had been affected by the whole cancer thing. I felt pressure to come up with a good answer. I made something up. We talked more about death and religion. Mike asked some pretty invasive questions. I think he is really struggling with his views in this area but I felt kind of used afterwards. He also said something which I felt troubling and which left me feeling angry towards him for the next couple of days. He said that it was hard for him to listen to some things we had to say about what was going on with me because he knew that things didn't always go well. When we told him how pleased our doctor was with my response to the first treatment, he thought to himself that this kind of response is not unusual and that the cancer still comes back. And even with the second treatment this can happen. He told me this as I'm going through my second treatment. I felt angry and afraid. I spent the next couple of days angry and afraid. I finally got over the anger and I talked to Mike about how I felt about what he said.

We are responsible for educating people on how
to treat us. And we are responsible for learning how
to treat other people.

≈≈

"They don't want to hear this," the doctor said to his young, dark-skinned intern, not even bothering to look at Bob or me while he spoke; he kept his pointy face with its salt-and-pepper beard turned away from us.

"But he has very little chance of surviving. Sure, I could pump him up with drugs and do a stem cell transplant, but that would only buy him a few months," he continued.

His announcement marked rock bottom arrival number three.

Speechless, too stunned to cause the uproar that this experience warranted we just sat there, immobile, rooted to our seats, our jaws on the cold linoleum floor.

Our oncologist had set up an appointment with this doctor to discuss a stem cell transplant. We were in no way prepared for what he was saying to us. No one had spoken to us so negatively about Bob's condition before this man. We knew his treatment was not going well, but we honestly just thought it was going to take a bit more effort than we had initially expected.

This man was the head of the transplant department and his presentation was insulting, degrading and infuriating, to say the least. He spoke as if we were not even in the room. His thin mouth casually spat out statistics as if Bob were not a real person sitting in front of him—as if he were a research subject.

Having just returned from our successful family reunion and vacation, we had felt very positive when we first walked into the office—jovial, even laughing. Annoyed by the two-hour wait, we were discussing how much patience we had learned over the last few months. We felt no sense of doom until this man had marched in the room, wearing a stiff white coat and round spectacles. Then the energy in the room shifted immediately, the air turned as cold and damp as if a blizzard wind had blown in.

We left the appointment in a daze, hardly able to comprehend the death sentence just handed to us. My heart pounded against my chest, desperate for escape. I looked up at Bob, his face blurry through the pool of tears standing in my eyes.

"Renie, OK, that wasn't good. But this thing isn't over," Bob said quietly.

He drew me to him. I buried my head in his shoulder, smelling the spicy scent of him, holding on so tightly, as if I could keep him with me by sheer force of will. I nodded mutely into his shoulder. *It can't be, it can't be,* ricocheted inside my head.

Focused on the emotional rather than the medical aspect of our current situation, I felt more outraged by our treatment than by the information itself. That doctor simply deflated us with his utter lack of human compassion.

We were incensed by the time we got to Kathy's to pick up Henry. Distracted, snacking on salty chips, we vowed never to return to that hospital. We were going to Nebraska to the transplant program there. A coworker of mine had been there with her husband for a successful bone marrow transplant, and they could not say enough good things about the place, describing it as if they spoke of their hometown.

Of course, all our anger was simply an attempt to distract ourselves from all-encompassing, bone-chilling terror.

Bob's journal
July 7, 2003

Today, Irene and I went to see the transplant guy, Dr. V. It was an awful experience. My heart was pounding two minutes after he started talking and never settled down. His message was that I have a very aggressive form of lymphoma and that at this point a stem cell transplant would not be successful. I have the option of trying another chemo regimen in the hopes that the cancer will respond to this and then do a stem cell transplant. He was very unencouraging that a new regimen would be successful. If it is not, he said the only recourse would be palliative.

We are crushed. I am still hopeful but this has been a difficult blow. I don't know how to respond emotionally.

≈≈

We arrived home after that appointment, and then the indignity of our mistreatment started to dissipate and the reality of the doctor's words began to sink in. I collapsed onto the ottoman in front of the fireplace, unable to take another step, and started to sob. I bent forward, rocking and wailing, a display I had not allowed myself until now. Bob knelt before me with his hands resting on my legs.

"I can't lose you, Bob. I can't raise two kids by myself. I can't. We should've gotten rid of this baby when we had the chance. We are so stupid. What an asshole," I bawled, shaking my head. My breath came in short bursts, and snot already clogged my nose. "You can't leave me, Bob. I can't do this without you. What am I going to do? I can't do any of this, you can't leave me alone here, I don't want to be doing this without you, I can't, I don't want to lose you," I pleaded with him, choking and gasping for breath.

Bob stayed right there in front of me as if trying to keep me from falling apart, limb from limb, right there in the living room. He didn't say a word, just remained there with me, his hands firmly on my thighs, a solid presence.

I don't know how long I carried on. It might have been quite a while or maybe just a moment. Slowly unfolding from the fetal position, coming back to my surroundings, my breathing slowing down, I looked around the dark room. My eyes landed on Henry on the other side of the room, quietly standing there and absorbing the entire scene, giving us the Henry Stare.

"Hey, Bud, do you want to watch *Blues Clues*?" I asked stupidly, attempting to distract him from this ugly scene. However, he was not a child who was easy to distract. He had straightforward questions that we answered as honestly as we could.

He knew that Daddy was sick and the doctors were trying to make him better. He knew the "straw" in Daddy's arm (Bob's PIC line) was how the medicine got in. He knew that because of that straw, Daddy was unable to go swimming with him that summer. He knew that the blood cancer Daddy had was so bad that the medicine they had to give him made his hair fall out. He knew he was staying with his aunts more often so that Mommy and Daddy could go to doctor appointments. He knew Mommy was having a baby.

He knew a lot, far more than any three-year-old should have to know. And now he knew that his mommy was terrified and that Daddy could get lost. How much more would he have to know before this was all done, I wondered?

Bob and I slowly stood up, parted, and began to resume normal action in the house. We moved about and started dinner; the house began to fill with the smell of garlic and onions. We had small talk and played with Henry, tried to normalize, and pretended that our world had not just been blown apart. That is what we did—we proceeded with the job before us because that was what we had to do. There were so many tasks before us that dealing with the ones right at hand was our only choice in that moment.

≈≈

We found ourselves back in the living room later, after getting Henry to bed in the usual fashion. This time I was sitting in Bob's La-Z-Boy chair, and he was on the floor. We were both lost in our own thoughts, gazing out at the living room and the blue Oriental rug, our tea growing cold beside us.

"I don't know, Renie. It just doesn't make sense to me; something is not right. What we have is so good." Bob looked up at me and motioned with his hands back and forth between us, as if drawing a line to connect us.

I got down on the floor to spoon with him on the scratchy rug. We spoke to each other. We spoke with honesty brought on by the waning light, by love, and by fear. We couldn't believe that we, Bob and Irene, could be over.

"Maybe we should sell the house. We could move in with my mom temporarily until we know what's going to happen," Bob said quietly.

I stiffened beside him. *He must believe what that doctor said.* Fear stabbed me in the chest. Bob sounded uncharacteristically defeated.

We left that suggestion hanging out there in the room, as if a fog were rolling in. We blew hot air at the damp mist, agreeing that we didn't feel like we could be over, not us.

What about all those conversations we'd had about when we were old and how we would be camping together in the Olympic National Forest? What about all the traveling we were going to do? What about all the experiences we planned for our children? The hikes and bike rides and family vacations and childhood milestones we anticipated?

"Our time will come again," was our mantra when we were feeling restricted by parenting. Now we had heard that it would not.

What about the fact that Bob had agreed to be the water parent? What about that? Was I now expected to get in the water with these two children on camping trips? I had to teach them to swim and to ride a bike? Oh, no, we had made a deal, and this wasn't the deal we'd made.

We lay there, and Bob felt so alive next to me, so warm and comforting, so vibrant, so secure, so *Bob*. What that doctor had said couldn't be true. We had just had the best sex of our lives the night before—really, a dying man wouldn't be doing that, would he? No, Bob wasn't dying. That idea was just ludicrous.

That doctor just didn't know Bob, and he didn't know us. He didn't know that Bob once climbed a mountain after vomiting earlier that morning. He didn't understand what kind of determination Bob had. He didn't understand how good we were together. He didn't know that early death wasn't supposed to happen to one of us.

He didn't know the plan.

≈≈

Bob's journal entries
July 11, 2003

Good news today. I had a CAT scan yesterday and the results were negative for any spreading to any areas other than the shoulder. Dr. Pierce came into my room chiming "I've got good news." I was immensely relieved. I think she was more certain of the result then I was. Afterwards she sent a couple of beers to my room to celebrate.

I feel like over the last week I have visited areas of my psyche that I never knew existed. I've gone from being ready to roll over and die to being determined to fight this thing to the very last breath. When I thought about death at one point there was almost a sweetness to it. Having to do with the cessation of all the complexities and demands of life. I think this is how I reconciled myself to what at that point I thought would be the almost certain outcome of this situation.

Cancer is forcing me to love life and to love life requires one to be very brave. It's also forcing me to rediscover aspects of myself which I have allowed to fall by the wayside as life's responsibilities have become more prominent.

Undated

Cancer is forcing me to be very bored and very sad and very lonely. It's Sunday morning and I've been in this damn hospital since Thursday morning—3 full days. A transplant will require me to be in the hospital for 3 weeks.

I've nothing to say or write about. I want to get out of here. I want to run away from this whole thing. I want to run away from the smells and the taste of this chemo. I want to run away from this pump. I want to run away from this hospital television. I want to run away from the sadness of what I still have to go through.

I'm tired. I'm tired of cycling through the stations on this TV.

July 21, 2003

I'm feeling relatively positive after a Monday spent mostly alone. I think I fear loneliness almost as much as the cancer these days. One thing Jim H. mentioned was the cancer should not be feared. It should be respected as a formidable enemy but not feared.

July 24, 2003

I want to beat this thing with every cell in my body. I want this as single mindedly as anything I have ever wanted. I am marshalling everything I have.

Today Henry left to go camping with his Aunts at the Stifter reunion. His birthday was yesterday and he got a purple bike from Jane and Larry.

Judy and the Highums prayed for me last night.

July 28, 2003

I'm tired. I'm tired of this whole cancer thing. I don't know how to address it with other people. I want to tell them I feel fine but that I worry, I'm afraid, I'm tired. It's been a long road and we still have a long way to go.

I feel anxious now. Physically I feel fine and intellectually I think that the course of treatment we have outlined is the right way to go.

> Cancer is a formidable foe. I feel confident that
> I am doing everything possible to win this battle.

≈≈

"My mom just introduced me to someone as 'my daughter Irene, the one whose husband has cancer.' Can you believe that?" I asked Bob, incredulous.

I was at my brother David's wedding in Montana. It was the beginning of August, three weeks and counting until Nebraska. Bob was at his sister's house so they could help him with Henry while I was away; the latest chemo had really knocked him on his ass.

I was talking on my sister's cell phone in the lobby outside the room where the reception was in full swing. I had to get away from the party, all the dancing bodies and tables of food. I had to talk to Bob.

"People keep saying how brave I am, Bob, as if we decided to get pregnant after your diagnosis or something. That wouldn't be brave. That would be stupid." I was babbling, of course, leaving Bob no time for response. I don't know if he was even awake on the other end. I don't know if it mattered.

"I'm not brave. What do these people know? Just because I am standing upright at this reception, does that make me brave? I would like to run screaming out of here and keep running, right past the airport. That is what I would like to do. What would people think then? I can't stand being here and watching all these people dance as if they don't have a care in the world. I can't answer another question about the stem cell transplant. I should be happy for my brother. They look so happy. I should be answering questions about how I am feeling. What about me? I am six months pregnant; does anyone want to talk about that?" I continued, hardly taking a breath.

"Oh, great," I said abruptly. "I have to go dance now. 'We Are Family' is playing." I could feel the unmistakable beat vibrating the floor beneath my feet. The hotel carpeting was a blur of red and gold. "I have to go dance with my sisters. Dance as if I am happy to be here!" I got ready to hang up, not even waiting for a reply.

"Renie, go dance with your sisters. I have to go throw up." Bob finally had a chance to talk.

Bob's journal entry
July 30, 2003

I am an old man and I have cancer. Can you believe it, fucking cancer. How could I, a seemingly simple, healthy, intelligent, boring, nondescript, Germanic, not too bright, cowardly, unaware, devious, demonic, industrious, noisy, loathsome, amazing, intricate, afraid of shadows and other insubstantial images—all this and I have cancer. So I am trying to do everything right. I am working hard. Staying up late trying to discover what combination of elements will defeat this enemy.

Irene suggests talking nicely and I have. I have talked sternly also. I have said, 'Give me my body back. This is my body. Give it back.' I will try anything. I have radically changed my diet. I've done three different kinds of chemo. I've done radiation, meditation, imagery. I'm doing counseling, trying to change my perception on life, lessen my fears, lower my anxiety, open my heart, be more authentic. Who am I really? Why am I jealous when others are happy? Why am I threatened by joy? How can I experience joy? How can I share my joy with others?

I lose myself in worry. How will we make it through this trial? Returning to work is a small worry but I feel that this job contributed to this illness. Maybe it didn't. I may have developed cancer regardless of my job or my emotional state. Do really happy people, fulfilled people get cancer? Probably. But this job is not contributing to my health.

My family, being limited in their involvement by distance, stepped up to the plate big time once the idea for a stem cell transplant in Nebraska became our latest plan. We barely had the OK from our insurance carrier and the doctors before my oldest sister, Anne, had found us an apartment and my parents had signed the short-term lease.

Anne called me with a proposed rotation of family members to come and go so we would never be there alone. Anne was always the organizer of the family. I am the youngest, born early on a Friday morning, and Anne and I were the only non-redheads of the siblings; we were bookends. Anne remained at home with the other five siblings while my parents went to the hospital to have me.

Anne, not yet eleven then, had taken her responsibility very seriously. When the neighbors stopped in to check on them, Anne assured them that everything was taken care of, announcing that they would stay home from school that day. She already had the others stripping their beds and cleaning up from the pancakes they had made for breakfast.

That was Anne's version of the morning.

My sister Colleen, number three, with bright red hair and a more restless nature, had a different memory. "Anne made us all stay home from school and do chores."

Anne was now suggesting we bring a blender to Nebraska because the apartment we would be staying in wouldn't have one. She remembered how important Henry's smoothie was to our morning routine.

I walked into the living room after hanging up the phone. Laughing, I repeated the conversation about the blender to Bob. I thought it was a cute story and very telling about the McGoldrick attention to detail.

Bob obviously did not find the story so funny. His eyes darkened with worry. I sat down, hands carefully placed on my knees, waiting for him to reveal himself.

"You know, Renie, I might not even be able to go to Nebraska. If my blood counts aren't good or if the radiation doesn't work …" he trailed off.

I appreciated his concern. It was not easy to be at the mercy of blood counts and doctors opinions. Now tickets were being purchased, calendars were being changed, and apartments were being rented—all this planning because of Bob. What if it didn't happen? What if we couldn't go? What if the tumor didn't go away?

"Well," I told him primly, "the McGoldricks are mobilizing, Bob. You can't stop them. This is their chance to help, to get involved. So we're going to Nebraska, whether or not you are getting a stem cell transplant—we are going to Nebraska."

I stood up and walked out of the room, without even a glance behind me.

Bob's journal entry
August 21, 2003

I'm paralyzed. We leave for Omaha on Tuesday and I feel like I have a long list of things I should be doing but I'm sitting around indecisively.

CHAPTER THREE

What About Nebraska?

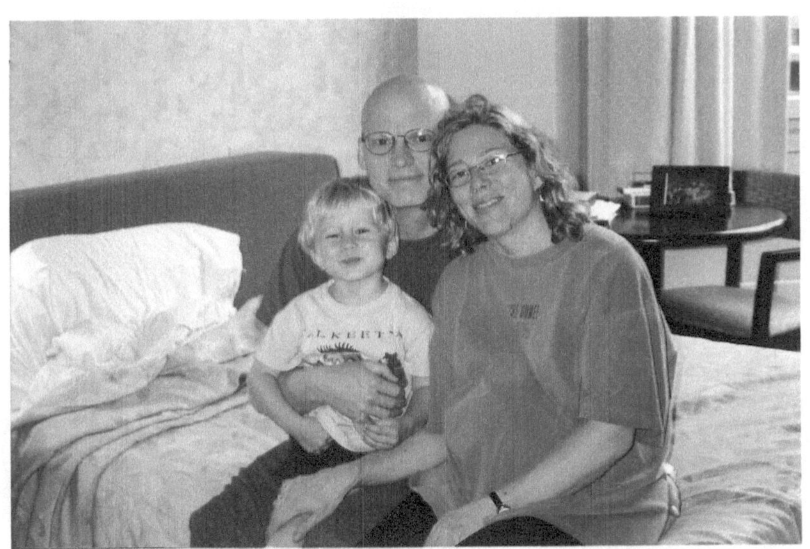

There must be dark and muddy waters
for the sun to background its shining glory.
Betty Smith, *A Tree Grows in Brooklyn*

<h2 style="text-align:center">Bob's journal entry
Aug 31, 2003</h2>

So we're in Omaha and I don't think I did many of those things I needed to do. I still need to make that list.

≈≈

"Don't vote for Bush," I heard my sister, Kathy, say as the rest of the sentence crackled in and out on our newly acquired cell phone. She was calling from the apartment in Nebraska that my parents had rented for us.

"Don't worry," I yelled back as I gingerly rocked my pregnant body back and forth, holding on to the gas pump for balance, trying to keep my face calm and my movements subtle. Sweat dripped idly between my shoulder blades. An RV blocked the sun as it maneuvered around the potholes to back up to a gas pump.

Kathy was first in the rotation of family members to stay with us in Nebraska. Her main job was to get to the apartment before 5:00 PM and secure the key. Because the current president was campaigning in her hometown, Dallas, Texas, at the time, all the flights from Dallas had been delayed.

"If not for the heroic driving of this Omaha cab driver, I wouldn't have made it in time," she explained breathlessly.

Still holding the phone, I waddled around the gas pump, shaking each leg until the searing pain running up each one subsided. The dense August heat was not helping my already swollen body as we sat in the car hour after hour, the sharp sting of hot asphalt drifting through the vents. Each pit stop was getting worse as the weight from my belly created too much pressure on the veins of my legs and made my blood pool in little pockets on the way back to my heart.

The three of us, Bob, Henry and I, were finally on our way to Nebraska, headed to the Lied Transplant Center on the University of Nebraska Medical Campus.

We were heading toward hope.

Watching the orderly rows of corn glide by, making big green waves in the fields along the highway, Bob and I contemplated our situation. Confused, we reminded each other how our oncologist, that first day in her office, had neatly organized Bob's care plan in outline and said "when" Bob was in remission, not "if".

Ideally, a person should be in remission before undergoing a stem cell transplant. We had anything but an ideal situation. No tactic or treatment had put Bob in remission. I would have done blood leeching at this point if someone had told me it would give Bob a few more years to live, just a few more years to be with his son and this new baby, due in another nine weeks.

Since his diagnosis just five months earlier, we had been through three different treatment plans, and the tumor on his shoulder just kept coming back, stronger, bolder, and angrier after each new chemo regimen—a most disrespectful tumor. He had undergone forty-five radiation treatments, and it was still too soon to know if the radiation had been successful at removing the tumor completely or had merely forced it into retreat to wait impatiently for its next strike.

We couldn't wait for the results; we needed to move while the tumor was at least in retreat.

As our desperation increased, so did our openness to try all avenues. Bob had recently submitted to being prayed over by his sister, Judy, and her family, an unlikely choice for him.

"Renie, I would piss on a radiator if I thought it would help," Bob politely responded to my question regarding his interest in the prayers.

Judy was the sibling closest in age to Bob, but light years away in her approach to life. Judy was more lighthearted, almost jolly, and seemed to wrap her arms around life and give it a big squeeze. She and her husband had four children and had been living in Atlanta for about twenty years.

Judy's family was what Bob and I referred to as fundamentalist Christian. Knowing Jesus and having him in their hearts were core family values preached regularly to us on visits in hopes of saving our souls. Their concern was genuine, but we found their attitude presumptuous.

Nevertheless, Bob sat serenely in the high-backed chair in the middle of the living room as if he were a king: I had resisted offering him some kind of staff. Henry and I sat on the couch while watching the scene unfold. Each member of the family walked up individually and touched Bob; each asked Jesus to shrink the tumor and remove the devil and any cancer cells from his body. Much of this came out so fast that I thought they all might have futures as auctioneers.

Henry sat motionless on my lap, taking it all in as I pondered the proceedings. *Do people who 'know' Jesus ever die from cancer?*

When their prayers were all done, Henry announced that he wanted to pray for Daddy too. All eyes on us, I assured him that if he wanted to pray for Daddy, he should. Henry remained still on the couch, looking at Bob and slowly blinking his insanely long lashes. None of us moved, waiting for him to take action.

"I'm done," he announced after some time.

I laughed to myself and gave him a little squeeze from behind in solidarity. *That's my boy, keeping his prayers to himself.*

≈≈

Wonderfully ignorant of the grueling procedure ahead, the three of us set off to Nebraska as if on an extended vacation. I had carried the bags out to the car, and Bob loaded them in, carefully placing the waffle iron next to the espresso machine. As I stumbled out the back door with the favorite pillows and blankets stacked under my chin, I glimpsed Bob wheeling out his bike; the rack was already on the car.

"We're going to have a lot of free time, Renie," Bob said quickly, seeing the doubtful look in my eyes. "I want to get Henry up on his new bike," he continued as he wheeled Henry's shiny purple bike out of the garage.

The bike was a gift from Aunt Jane for Henry's third birthday, and he was thrilled. Henry perfected braking that very first night; he enjoyed slamming on the brakes at the last minute, just before he careened into the middle of an uncontrolled intersection. Unable to chase after him due to my basketball belly, I had to trust that Henry knew what he was doing.

Bob motioned toward my bike with his head, and I peered into the garage, where my poor bike waited, all alone. Thinking about my knees hitting my belly on each upswing of the pedal, I shook my head. Best to leave the biking to the boys on this trip.

≈≈

The three of us arrived at the apartment in Omaha at dusk, sticky from the heat and exhausted from the continual buzz of anxiety that had stayed with us since Bob's diagnosis. We pulled into an apartment complex like any apartment complex, a half dozen buildings two stories high, with some walkways connecting the buildings. Young trees were planted along the green spaces. Once in the lobby, Henry spied the elevator and immediately thought this was the coolest place ever. The elevator led to a hallway that led to generic one- and two-bedroom apartments. Laundry facilities were down the hall.

Kathy led us to the pool immediately, a life-saving benefit of the apartment complex. Standing in front of the mirror while putting my suit on, I thought the cold damp tiles beneath my feet were somewhat refreshing, but the smell of Lemon Pledge was so thick that it got caught in my throat. I leaned on the sink and stood on my left foot while I guided my right foot into my suit. Then I noticed what appeared to be a growth high up on the inside of my thigh, creeping up towards the elastic on my swimsuit like a caterpillar on steroids.

There they were, the dreaded varicose veins that my mother had warned me about—the car ride had proven too much for my weak veins.

"Ah, boy," I moaned softly. I thought varicose veins only happened on legs; I never expected them *there. How am I supposed to birth a baby? I might pop something vital.* I mused.

Varicose veins seemed low on the roster of concerns that night, so I kept the unfortunate development to myself and simply savored the moment as I slid into that cool water. Breathing deeply, filling my ribcage slowly as my body became weightless, I relaxed, leaned my head back for a moment and floated, letting the water cradle me under the creamy August moon.

≈≈

Day one in Omaha was busy. Kathy dropped Bob and me off at the circle drive of the Lied Transplant Center, a beige, nondescript twelve-story building that stands taller than any other building on the medical campus. This structure is a beacon of hope and expectation for cancer patients in need of transplants.

At the busy entrance, I watched carefully as family members wheeled their loved ones out of the building and toward their packed cars. One could conjure up visions of moving day at a college dorm. As Bob and I walked past the suitcases and parked wheelchairs, I tried to sneak a glimpse at people's eyes and maybe glimpse my future. Did their eyes hold fear, resignation, anticipation?

Bob and I sat at one end of the table in the nurses' office. This session was meeting number four or five of the back-to-back meetings with all the professionals we would be dealing with throughout the stem cell transplant procedure. This one was dressed in casual business attire and sounded a bit blasé about the information she was presenting to us from the other side of the table. No bells or whistles or whoops of delight sounded as she explained how this miracle of modern science would work. She just kept pointing out charts and lists and sliding paperwork towards us. Reluctantly I reached for each new sheet, adding it to the growing stack. Maybe she was tired of couples like us, naïve and trusting, counting on this treatment to be their magic bullet.

"Do you have any questions?" she finally asked with a forced smile, coming to the end of her presentation.

Bob was prepared with the same questions he had asked each time someone asked us that one.

"Yeah," he responded, clearing his throat and pulling his chair closer to the table and getting his pen ready. "Are there any good bike trails nearby?" Then he asked, "Where do you purchase the best organic produce in town?"

Caught off guard initially, the nurses, social worker, and dietician were eventually able to come up with quite a few suggestions for us. Bob and I walked out of the Lied Transplant Center that first day with a list of bike trails, parks, activities, and organic food stores in Bob's spiral notebook. This notebook was the place where hope met desire. The entries were a wish list of possibilities.

I was loaded down with the three-ring binder with "Lied Transplant Center" stamped boldly on the front. This binder was where hope met reality, each entry a piece of fact. Everything we needed to survive the next seven weeks of our life was in this binder—all the names and the numbers and the instructions and the procedures and the appointments and the dates.

≈≈

Bob's journal entry
August 31, 2003

I met this guy, B., today. He's a cabinet maker from Minnesota. He just had an allogenic mini-transplant. He told me his diagnosis and it's almost exactly the same as mine. This freaked me out a little bit because he said he had a stem cell transplant like the one I'm getting and he went into remission for a year but then his cancer came back. I don't want this cancer to come back. I want to be done with this shit now.

≈≈

Morning number two came, and Bob woke up with a fever. We also found that the apartment had no running water. I sat on the couch in the dent his hips made as he lay curled up there. The two of us quietly discussed our best course of action. Chuckling nervously, we tried not to interrupt my sister Kathy's tirade on the phone.

"We have a man with cancer here, a pregnant woman, and a three-year-old. We need the water turned back on! Is there a manager I can talk to? Excuse me … what …."

"He hung up on me! Can you believe that? I am calling him back—that is unbelievable. That was uncalled for, don't you think? This is unacceptable!" Kathy picked up the phone again and pounded the number into the keypad, her face flushed from indignation.

"I hope you don't get us a pink slip," I joked, wanting to lighten the situation.

In our big picture, considering what we were doing here and the fact that Bob was a fevered blob next to me, the lack of running water was not high on my priority list at the moment. Someone should be worried about running water, though, and Kathy was taking her job very seriously. The color of her face was matching the red in her hair.

It turned out that Bob had developed a bacterial infection and required a four-day infusion of antibiotics to combat the little devils. These infusions were not a good way to begin our Nebraska adventure, putting our tight time schedule in peril right from the start. I felt catapulted into the rhythm of the clinic, its beat different from all others. Time did not have the same meaning as the outside world; it was measured by lab results and treatment schedules, not the numbers on the clock or dates on a calendar.

≈≈

Bob's journal entry
September 2002

It would have been the first day of the school year for me today. I'm not sorry I'm missing it. I am incredibly unsatisfied with my chosen profession at the moment. I have never really found a work environment that I have loved. I'm always envious of people who have found a profession they enjoy. It seems like an almost miraculous thing. I can only imagine what it must be like.

The whole thing troubles me quite a bit because I clearly don't want to keep doing something I don't enjoy. The problem is I can't conceive of anything I would enjoy doing.

I'm bored. I'm boring. I, I, I.

Brain is no longer functioning.

Just want to get out of here and ride bike through forest trail, jump off cliff into sky blue waters. Drink beer around a camp fire with friends. Canoe down a river rapidly. Christmas dinner, ham, mashed potatoes.

≈≈

Bob was receiving an autogenic or "auto" stem cell transplant, meaning he was harvesting his own stem cells, as opposed to an allogenic, or "allo", as it is known at the transplant center, which is from a donor.

The agenda of the transplant was to harvest Bob's stem cells, load him up with high doses of chemo to kill off any cancer cells lingering in his body, and then infuse him with the stem cells that would allow his body a fresh start to rebuild his immune system.

The stem cell transplant was an oil change for the lymph system, to steal a phrase from our friend and fellow transplant survivor, Jim.

The most compelling and enduring reason we picked the Lied Transplant Center was because of its Cooperative Care Program. Cooperative Care (co-op) is a unique approach to health care delivery that allows a family member to be the care partner during the entire treatment process.

The Lied Transplant Center is the only oncology unit designed with cooperative care in mind. Participants stay in hotel-like rooms complete with a sitting area separated from the rest of the suite by French doors. The rooms are just an elevator ride away from the treatment center, a workout area, a computer/library room, and a playroom for children. Every room has a kitchenette, and there is a dining room down the hall in the hospital. Cooperative Care Program patients get a punch card to obtain meals and snacks there.

I was immediately drawn to the concept of cooperative care. Since the grape incident, as we now kindly referred to it, and Bob's neglect in telling me about the first recurrence, I obsessively wanted to be closely involved in the process Bob was experiencing. Cooperative care put me right in the middle of all the action.

We expected to be in Omaha for seven weeks. That meant arriving two weeks prior to the transplant for training and harvesting, four weeks in the co-op, and a week after discharge for monitoring before we could return home.

The process was very structured, with every day numbered. The first official day of the transplant regimen is called day minus six. On day zero, the medical team infuses the new stem cells into the patient. On days seven through nine, the recipient "bottoms out". That means that his white blood cell count is at zero; he essentially has no immune system. By days eleven through thirteen, the stem cells are starting to reattach and produce some white cells, and the recipient should begin to improve. At day twenty-one, the patient should be ready for discharge from the co-op.

≈≈

Once we got Bob's initial infection cleared up, we began the training needed for me to care properly for Bob throughout the ordeal. I would be responsible for taking his vitals (blood pressure, temperature, and other checks) and recording them; monitoring self-medication; performing daily blood draws; transporting Bob to and from treatments; doing dressing changes; flushing his central line; and reporting any changes to the nurse.

Sitting in a room with a few other couples, we were surrounded by gauze, latex gloves, masks, syringes, tubing, alcohol wipes, and the other paraphernalia needed to change the dressing covering the central line safely. The line had been surgically placed in Bob's chest after we arrived in Omaha, replacing the PIC line in his arm.

Half joking that I might kill him, imagining air bubbles traveling through his veins, I concentrated on tapping the air out of the saline I had just drawn into the syringe.

"I'm as good as dead," Bob teased as I clumsily attempted to secure the tape around the gauze. Studying the written instructions placed neatly on the desk, I took a deep breath, trying to get my nervous laughter under control, but little chortles and hiccups kept escaping. Were we bothering the other couples as they attempted to concentrate on these tasks? Was the instructor looking annoyed? Worried? Every group had to have one couple like us in it, right?

When Bob and I were pregnant with Henry, we took the ten-part Bradley Method (natural birth) birthing classes. We never took the exercises as seriously as our instructor had hoped we would. I would lie obediently on my side, curled up in the fetal position, part on and part off the oriental rug in the middle of her living room. I was never sure if the rug smelled like stale farts or if it was only the power of suggestion from the regular eruptions from our instructor while she spoke to us about the opening of the cervix and the evils of epidurals. The force of her gas raised her little body up a bit to one side, and the sound of its escape echoed against the wood floor. It was all the rest of us could do to keep our faces straight.

Bob would wrap one arm around me and rub my lower back with the other as he supposedly whispered to me our mantra that would take me to my happy place during a contraction. Having not discussed the mantra, he would instead whisper to me about where we should go to dinner after class.

"Kopps has mint chocolate chip custard today," he whispered seductively into my ear, tickling the lobe a little and starting me on a giggling jag.

"I assure you, you won't be laughing during a contraction when you're really in labor," the instructor reprimanded us in her nasal voice and knowing tone.

"We'll show her," we assured ourselves on the way home as we made our way through the dark streets of the lakefront neighborhood, looking at the brick turn-of-the-century estates, then illuminated by a single street lamp.

Well, we got through the birth with no problems, and we even laughed a few times. We could do this transplant thing too, I hoped, as I continued to study the instruction sheet.

≈≈

Initially our time in Omaha was an odd juxtaposition of events. The vacation feeling lingered, even amongst all the appointments and incisions and trainings for this life-threatening/life-giving procedure.

We were in a new city; it was early fall, and the air was still warm but no longer stagnant. There were sounds of crunching leaves and afternoon football games. We had family members helping us, all those chores at home seemed far away, and our priorities were clear. We stocked the apartment with organic food and discovered a nice walking trail close by the apartment. There were new coffee shops to visit and restaurants to discover.

Henry was able to satisfy his unending biking jones at the parking lot across from the apartment. We waited for the last stragglers to leave work before we all trooped across the street so Henry could cruise around the open lot in the fading summer light, heading straight for each median, furiously braking before hurtling himself into a crabapple tree. Bob and I were used to these antics by now, but my sister Anne lost years of her life on that blacktop.

≈≈

Anne was number two in the rotation. Anne, the oldest, left for college when I was seven and essentially never returned. She married and started her family while young. My mom has always given Anne credit for raising me those early years, and I was devastated when she left for college. As the story goes, I kissed her high school picture on the mantel every night before I went to bed.

Time passed, and we became very different people. The different choices that Anne and I made in our twenties made our age difference seem wider. We didn't live in the same state most of the time and were each absorbed in our own lives. Anne raised a family of three boys on a shoestring budget and a glass-half-full disposition. Meanwhile, I moved and traveled and went to school, carrying my more cynical outlook throughout it all.

Once on a family reunion in Ireland, while still childless, I overheard a conversation between Anne and her oldest son. He was nineteen at the time, and he had been a serious and studious child from the beginning. The entire family was embarking on a two-day venture to the Aran Islands, and Anne was telling him what he should pack, down to the underwear he would need. He merely nodded as he secured his bag from the trunk of the van.

"He's nineteen, I think he can handle how many pairs of underwear to bring on an overnight trip," I said later to Bob.

On that same trip, Bob and I shared a minivan with Anne and her husband, Scott, a musician by passion and a salesman by trade. I asked Scott if he ever questioned Anne's directives.

"Why should I?" he responded with a contented shrug. While my parents, in the front seat, noisily negotiated the roundabouts and Gaelic street signs, Scott continued evenly, saying, "Everything's always turned out so far."

I shrugged back and smiled smugly, believing I knew more about independence and freedom than he did.

≈≈

"Anne's going to be with us for eleven days, Bob," I had commented one evening as we prepared for our trip to Nebraska. We had just received the proposed McGoldrick family rotation.

"What on Earth will we talk about?" I couldn't fathom how we'd have enough in common to last that many days.

Well, after eleven days with Anne, I was singing a new tune. What *didn't* we talk about? We talked nonstop. We reconnected as sisters should—unconditionally.

One morning Anne and I sat at the dining room table. My frothy chai steamed next to us. Bob had already gone to one appointment or the other. Henry gripped his sippy cup of smoothie in one hand as he snaked a train track throughout the apartment, brightening up the bland carpet with the blue and red trains. Anne pulled out a piece of paper and pencil, straightened her chair and her back, and smoothed her hair behind her ears—her list-making position.

"I thought I'd go to the grocery store," she said, as if talking to herself while I just happened to be present, "and buy stuff for the week. Now, Mom and Dad will be here at the end of the week, so I thought we could make meat loaf and freeze it so there will be an easy meal when they arrive."

Was I supposed to be paying attention? Did she ask me something? Is today the day I change Bob's dressing, or does the tubing just need flushing? When should Bob be home from the center today? Was he just getting the shot today?

"Do you like beef stroganoff?" Anne continued seamlessly. "With the leftover meat, I thought we could make some beef stroganoff for us tonight. My kids always liked that." She stood up and purposefully began to clear the breakfast dishes and load the dishwasher.

"How does that sound?" she stated rather than asked, glancing at me over the bar that separated the kitchen from the dining room. "I will throw in a load of laundry on our way out. Henry, let's get your teeth brushed. We're leaving." Henry put the train down and walked to the bathroom as if brushing his teeth was his only option.

All I could do was lean on the table as if for support and watch the scene before me, vaguely realizing that I did not command that kind of authority with Henry. Desiring to absorb Anne's parenting style by osmosis, my mind kept wandering. *My OB appointment is tomorrow, right?* I pondered as I continued to watch Henry prepare to get in the car. *Yes, tomorrow ... I will walk over there while Bob is doing the harvesting ... he starts the harvesting tomorrow ... I wonder how long that will take? I am thirty-two weeks now ... I would like to be home by thirty-seven weeks ... if it takes him three days to harvest, what we need ...*

"Beef stroganoff? That sounds yummy," I stated abruptly. "Shopping? Great, that sounds good. OK, we're leaving. Where's Henry?" I attempted to move the present moment into the forefront, envisioning the tape reel in my forehead moving around the side of my head, above my ears and into the back of my head. There it sat, trapped and lurking, the weeks ticking by, unheeded.

I never felt oppressed by Anne's authority, which she conveyed through presentation of facts. She would state the details in a way that did not necessitate a decision on my part, yet implied that I could weigh in if I so chose. While my mind was crowded with transplant details, the week was mapped out for us, the activities of daily living managed. Bob and I had agreed that if our situation got bad and we needed help, we would call on Anne. We had seen firsthand what her family knew all along.

For both Bob and me, Anne was an unexpected present in our stocking full of coal.

≈≈

While Anne was in Omaha to perform her magic with Henry, I took a brief, impractical, trip to Colorado for a high school friend's wedding. What I wanted most from this trip was a chance to pretend I led a normal life, not talk about cancer and stem cells and doctor appointments for thirty-six hours, and simply witness another person's joy.

So I stood there at the reception, alone among the crowd in the thin, cool evening air, and watched as my friend, looking very regal and tall in her elegant ivory dress, gave a beautiful toast. I tried, for all the world, to feel as if nothing else mattered in this moment. Then an unexpected mention of Bob in the bride's toast and unfamiliar arms around my shoulders in comfort brought me back to the reality of my life. I had to stifle the sudden urge to scream about the naïveté of everyone in the room. Did anyone here really know the meaning of "in sickness and in health"?

≈≈

"It's all about Bob. Everything is all about Bob. No one cares that I'm pregnant. Everywhere I go, it's all about Bob." The words crackled and popped across the table at lunch the day following the wedding. I was with my friend, Margaret, and my sister-in-law, Kate.

Margaret and I had been friends since we were in the sixth grade. We had been little gymnasts together and spent many afternoons stuffing our faces with French fries at the Tastee Freeze before going to the gym to practice back handsprings on the beam. I had always been so envious of her dark hair, spending most of our college years telling her how good that sweater or that blouse looked against the dark contrast of her hair and eyes.

Margaret and I had our practical ways in common. However, I thought that Margaret, like most of my friends, was much nicer than I was. She and I had lived together in college, spent a summer in a one-bedroom cottage with four girls on Cape Cod, and traveled to Europe together after college. There was little I could say that would surprise Margaret.

But I think I might have done it that afternoon; all I could hear was the clinking of china and glasses, the breeze from the waitstaff as they hurried by, the murmur of voices from the tables around us, the occasional burst of laughter from across the room. Utter silence came from across the table. Two sets of brown eyes stared back at me.

"I told Bob, 'Fine, you have your year. But next year is mine. Next year it's all about Irene.'" The waiter filled our water glasses, removed our plates, and tried to avert his eyes.

≈≈

Back at our Nebraska apartment, Anne turned down the volume on the *Thomas the Tank Engine* video while I grabbed for the phone. The three of us were killing time while waiting for Bob to return from his doctor appointment. He had completed his first day of harvesting, and we were anxious for a report on how it had gone.

"woo hoo," I cheered. My hands went up in the air in the universal sign for victory. "It seems as though Bob is a super producer!" I excitedly announced to Anne and Henry after I hung up the phone.

Bob had collected enough stem cells the very first day! We had been told that this fact meant nothing regarding the outcome of the transplant, but there was much elation in the apartment anyway. We had to celebrate the little victories. We believed it had to indicate something good; it couldn't be bad.

Bob was strong and feeling better than he had in months. I figured that anyone who would ride a bike to harvest his stem cells had to be ok. If nothing else, we made up some days on our timeline for the return to Milwaukee. We were back on schedule now.

Bob's treatment just might go according to plan. I might not have to give birth to a Cornhusker.

≈≈

Anne, Henry, and I went to the mall for a change of scenery one afternoon. Henry was laughing and jumping and having a wonderful time in a ball pit until his blonde head popped up from beneath the multicolored plastic balls. His face scrunched up, and he started screaming. He had twisted his foot. Henry was usually rather stoic about injuries, but this time he carried on and on and wouldn't put any weight on it as we made our way to the car.

Anne thought we might want to bring him to the hospital and have it looked at.

"I cannot deal with another hospital and more doctors. I just can't. We'd have to wait and ..." Panic was starting to rise toward my throat. I could taste the familiar tinny flavor of fear. "What would they tell us anyway? Elevate and ice it, right?" I declined, shaking my head and crossing my arms like a petulant child.

Anne quietly drove us to the health food store so I could read through the essential oils book and see what oils were suggested to speed healing and help with swelling. I had been relying on the healing properties of essential oils since we lived in Portland, rarely using more common medications. The irony of Bob and myself, both minimal medication users, being in a situation where the granddaddy of all medication was being used, was not lost on us.

Birch oil was said to be good for bone healing and inflammation. The only essential oils I had brought with us were tea tree and lavender, which I considered my desert island oils, both good to ward off infections. The closest I could find at the store was cypress oil; it was supposed to aid with circulation, and it was from a tree. I hoped that if I used it with the intention to heal the bone, it would work. Anne was skeptical and convinced me to purchase some baby aspirin on the way home for the pain.

The next morning was the true test. Would Henry remember he was injured at all? Henry jumped out of bed and began howling. If he had forgotten, he was quickly reminded when he tried to put weight on his foot.

"Hmmmmmm," Bob and I mumbled to each other from across the hall. Maybe this injury was serious.

We will never know. Bob and I successfully denied the issue; the thought of another health crisis in our family proved too much for our battered psyches. After a few days of elevating and icing and dropping cypress and lavender oil on Henry's foot, the swelling came down, the purple and yellow bruises started to fade, and his limping diminished.

The entire incident faded into the background of chemotherapy and blood counts rather quickly.

≈≈

Move-in day at the co-op arrived.

There had also been a changing of the guard. My parents arrived for their shift and had taken Anne to the airport. I was too distracted to miss her; family members seemed to float in and out seamlessly. Bob's sisters and mom and a friend were there at one point, then my sisters and parents, then Bob's brother, Eugene. I wanted to spend more time with each one, but there was always another one to see.

The time felt a bit like a long-drawn family reunion (or memorial service).

Bob and I watched as his sisters pulled away in Jane's little SUV and headed off on their eight-hour driving adventure with Henry, who was secured in his car seat. They were taking him for three weeks while we were "checked in". The big electric door slowly closed behind them, leaving us in the dark and damp underground garage. We walked past the row of parked cars toward the elevator, pushed the button for floor seven, and continued down the hall to our room.

Paper cranes greeted us the instant we opened the door. Stuffed in every nook and cranny were big cranes, small cranes, yellow cranes, red cranes. Cranes were in the drawers and on the shelves above the TV, under both beds, under the sink in the kitchenette. My sister, Teri, and her family knew of a Japanese fable that maintains that if a person sees a thousand cranes, he gets his wish. So she and her two grade-school children hand-made a thousand origami cranes, folding like crazy at baseball games and during their long drives down the canyon from their home in Estes Park to Boulder or Denver. My parents were charged with transporting the cranes in their car from Colorado and had distributed them throughout our room while we said our stilted good-byes to Henry.

Could there have been a miscount? Did one get lost in transit?

≈≈

Bob's journal entry
September 13, 2003

Today is the third day of chemo and I'm still feeling pretty strong. I still have three days of chemo to go and then the transplant will be Wednesday. After that it's all recovery.

Henry left today with Kathy and Jane. Irene's parents are here staying at the apartment and I'd been wondering why we didn't just keep Henry at the apartment with them but I guess considering the shape I'm going to be in over the next couple of weeks, it's probably a good thing he won't be here. I think it would have been a beneficial thing for him to spend more time with Dave and Nancy. I would have liked for that to happen.

I'm seeing a therapist here but I don't really feel like I'm getting anything accomplished. I don't know whether to dig up ancient history or focus on current issues.

I think my two big issues are aloneness and not meeting expectations. This not meeting expectations is the interesting one. I'm not sure how the two are tied together but around most other adults I don't feel like an adult. I don't feel as well-informed or as connected or as competent as I should be. I'm not a doctor or a lawyer or an artist or someone with a true passion for any particular thing. I'm not a person who has cultivated interests. I don't know much about anything this is how I usually feel around other adults. I feel less significant. So, whose standards am I not living up to?

Why do I continually play this comparison game in which I almost invariably come up short.

Is it my height? Is it because I am too short? What if I were a big, tall, burly strong man with a beard and fiery red hair. Then would I be adequate? Then would I be satisfactory? What if I were very organized and charismatic, a leader of men, brimming with solutions to all the world's ills? What if I were gregarious and charming, filled with energy and enthusiasm? Then would I be adequate? What if I had not given up on myself?

So how can I reorient this whole thing? How can I start to see myself apart from other people and as adequate in my own right? Is it just

affirmations—I'm good enough, I'm strong enough
and gosh darnit …? Is it awareness of these feelings?
Is there a third choice in addition to either superior
or inferior.…

≈≈

"I feel like this is our second honeymoon," I chuckled to my dad,
half seriously, as we walked down the seafoam-green hallway. The
color was chosen to be calming, I am sure, and we were on our way
from the dining room to our room in the co-op one evening.

For the present, I had no child or household responsibilities, a
nice hotel room, and food provided. All we needed was a Jacuzzi
bath, and we would be set.

A second honeymoon with chemo?

≈≈

September 17, 2003, arrived—Bob's re-birthday, day zero. The
staff in the clinic, dressed in their scrubs, were in a flurry of activity
as they set up the infusion. They were efficient yet casual, as if this
were not the most momentous occasion of our lives.

I had expected the kind of buzz there is in a room when a baby
is born, that electric energy that makes a person feel anything is
possible. This energy was more cautious, a bit yearning. The air
smelled tangy, as if fear were mixed with an alcohol rub. My parents
and I attempted small talk about the election and the status of the
Cubs as we perched on the chairs surrounding Bob, who semireclined
in the La-Z-Boy. Our eyes moved between Bob, the nurses, and the
nurses' station, placed strategically in the middle of the circle of
treatment rooms, separated by sliding glass doors. The nurses hung
bright red bags filled with stem cells to IV poles and attached the
tubing to his central line.

At first Bob dropped one-liners into our conversation between
pokes and sticks with needles and thermometers. Eventually his head
sagged to the side as the Benadryl used to counteract an allergic
reaction took effect. Our conversation went on around him.

I felt like I had icicles stabbing me every time I took a breath. I felt distant from the events going on around Bob and me. Then I inhaled sharply, involuntarily, and there was a shift in my chest, as if the sharp edges had melted away. I felt that old comfortable blanket, Bob's presence, surround me. Without realizing that it had been gone, I now felt utter relief to have it back.

We had been orbiting each other emotionally, like the moon and the sun, reliant on each other's patterns, but never in the same place at the same time. Each of us had been fighting our own battle and exhausting our resources in the process.

Lying in that reclining chair with fresh stem cells being infused into his blood stream, Bob surrendered what energy he could spare. He handed over his weighted, grounding energy to calm my jittery, overactive mind. I would need both his energy and my own to get through these next few weeks.

In no time we were back in our room, a bit dazed, as if we had woken up from a nap and weren't sure if it was the next day or not. Unsure of what to do next, we could only wait. Watching numbers, blood counts, temperatures, and blood pressures, we waited.

≈≈

In the co-op, we found a camaraderie like that in a college dorm. We would ride the elevator together to the treatment center, talk or wave in the cafeteria, remove dry clothes from the drier, and place them on top of it to make room for our own wet clothes.

We would see a subtle nod of commiseration as we pushed our ailing loved ones down the hall. I couldn't help comparing Bob's appearance to that of the other patients—that guy was paler, that gal was thinner, that guy's wife looked tired. There was a lot of talk about what day each patient was on. I was always trying to see what we had in store; what did people look like on day nine or eleven or fifteen?

Each morning I would need to secure one of three blood pressure machines so I could get Bob's vitals before going down for rounds with the doctors at 8:00 AM. If I was lucky enough to find one of them standing in the hallway, I would dash down the hall, glancing behind me to see if anyone might be making a move on it. I would grab it and wheel it back to the room as if I were looting.

≈≈

The two of us waited every morning in the treatment room for the doctors to come and tell us the results of the daily blood draw. The results would shape the rest of our day. What would his white blood cell count be? What about his platelets, his potassium?

"What restaurant do you want to go to first when we get back home?" I asked Bob as I sat down next to him and pulled out my daily Krispy Kreme doughnut, which I washed down with a Dr. Pepper. Both items came from the cafeteria and felt rather like contraband. The poor baby! When I was pregnant with Henry, I'd eaten only nuts and berries.

Bob tried to be a good sport. "Nothing sounds good right now. Maybe we could go get that red curry you like so much on the east side."

I licked the jelly from my fingers and sucked the dark liquid from the straw as if it were bootleg whiskey. Bob surfed the TV channels for the hundredth time that morning. Our eyes mostly looked through the sliding panes of glass that separated us from the nurses' station. All the treatment rooms faced inward in a circle around the nurses' station. We could watch them as they prepared the meds and syringes and bags of various fluids and gossiped amongst themselves. We tried to read their lips, wondering if they were talking about us.

Eventually the team of doctors would file in and linger in the doorway in their long white coats and stethoscopes. They held their clipboards exactly the way a Jehovah's Witness clutches a Bible while standing on your doorstep—with reverence and just a little fear. All of them had their eyes on the chart while the lead doctor came all the way in the room and shook Bob's hand.

"How are you today, Mr. Wellenstein?" He or she would open with the basic pleasantries. "Love your pants." Many of the doctors commented on Bob's "fishy pants", as we referred to them. We bought them at a yard sale Sarah and Garrett had just before we left for Nebraska. They were fleece and had large neon-colored fish all over them, and Bob wore them nearly every day of our stay. They made quite a splash at the center.

"What day are we on?" was always one of the first questions. They weren't really asking us. They were thinking aloud as they interpreted the information in front of them.

They would tell us the story of Bob's blood, and we anxiously waited for the tale to be told. The two of us watched his white blood cells drop every day, reading the daily report as if we were stockbrokers during a depression, desperate for the numbers to bottom out so they could start the slow climb back up.

Initially Bob appeared unchanged, but by day four, he had lost his appetite, developed a bacterial infection, and his potassium was low. These were not uncommon complications, the staff explained. They had a remedy for each dilemma——shots, infusions, and an enormous pill for the low potassium.

Day eight was the ten-year anniversary of our first date. My parents were sent on a mission to find the movie we had seen that night. They arrived at our room with *The Wedding Banquet* proudly in hand. Bob and I attempted to curl up on the hospital bed, my belly and Bob's IV pole unwelcome guests at this long-anticipated celebration. Bob was asleep ten minutes into the subtitled movie.

I muted the movie and spent the rest of the gloomy evening with silent, flashing pictures from the TV falling over both of us. Bob was up and down, going between bed and bathroom. I watched him struggle to muster the energy required to propel his body out of bed. He muttered in disgust. His shoulders were hunched, but his steps remained determined as he made his way across the room.

My mind drifted to our courtship and the way Bob's body felt when I wrapped my arms around him and laid my cheek to his shoulder when he took me for a spin on his motorcycle. His chest was strong but yielding during the exhilaration of the ride.

When was the last time that we held each other and I felt that composed strength? The protective shield that came around us during the transfusion and softened my reality was disintegrating fast. The room came into exaggerated focus and seemed to pulse with intensity. Wherever I looked, I saw reminders of why we were here—gauze, latex gloves, pill boxes.

The honeymoon was over.

≈≈

By day nine or ten, he began staggering to the bathroom while gripping his IV pole for balance. Bob refused my help with a wave of his hand, and I sat upright on the edge of the bed and watched. My heart pounded in my chest, my breath was shallow, and I was ready to pounce. I was hoping, hoping, hoping that I would not have to pick him up off the floor.

The evening nurse visited each co-op room and brought a medication box for the next twenty-four hours. It was reassuring to have a professional come once a day and look over the vital entries and monitor our situation. We asked her questions regarding Bob's lack of appetite and strength, and she offered suggestions and comfort, gentle assurance that what he experienced was expected in these circumstances. Rarely does a person sail through recovery without an issue.

≈≈

Finishing up our third Scrabble game of the day, my parents and I contemplated lunch ideas. I glanced at Bob's inert body lying on the other side of the French doors and hesitated.

"I'll stay here, Renie Boo, you and your mom go get a bite to eat," my dad suggested.

Thankful for the respite, I ran out the door and didn't look back.

"Renie, you gotta get your dad to stop hovering," Bob complained later that evening, after my parents had gone back to the apartment.

"I know it can be annoying, but they are here to help. They need to help," I tried to explain.

"Well, I need to be left alone. I don't need hovering, and I don't like your parents seeing me like this," he insisted.

"Bob, they are here for me, not you. I need them here. I need them, so you have to deal." I know I sounded heartless about his legitimate need for privacy, but in that moment I didn't care. I was sinking under the weight of the responsibility, and my parents offered a life jacket. I never refuse a life jacket.

≈≈

By day twelve or so, Bob was dangerously low on platelets, but none were available immediately. We learned that a direct donation from a specific donor could be arranged, and my mom graciously volunteered. In the end, after eating a pound of raisins to increase her iron levels, she was unable to collect the platelets, blowing out her own vein in the attempt.

Then it was day fourteen, maybe, and Bob's blood pressure was low. Bags of saline were given through his IV. The evening nurse requested that Bob come to the clinic for blood pressure monitoring, and an offer was made that Bob stay in the clinic that night.

I jumped at the chance for time off. I wasn't sleeping, and that was not just because of Bob, but because the baby would get the hiccups every night. The gentle nudges in my belly were aggravating. I longed for a swift kick in the ribs.

I knew we were dangerously close to being transferred to the inpatient transplant wing of the hospital. If a patient requires more than eighteen hours out of twenty-four in the treatment room, that patient is supposed to go to the inpatient hospital. I interpreted "going inpatient" as a failure on my part to meet Bob's needs as his care partner.

I understood that of the patients who start in the co-op, 90 percent stay in the co-op the whole time. I did not want to be part of the other 10 percent, seeing it as a bad omen for the outcome of the transplant.

While down in the clinic that evening, still waiting for the platelets, Bob tripped over his tubing on the way to the bathroom.

"What in the hell happened, Bob?" I cried, seeing him lying in the darkened clinic room the next morning. He looked as if someone had beaten him up. He had a big gash on his forehead, not an ideal situation when one is low on platelets.

The staff resorted to my pregnancy as an argument for inpatient care.

"Look, I'm fine. This baby is the safest one among us, so don't try using this baby as an excuse. I can do this. I've been doing this. We can do this!" Proud of my advocacy skills, I repeated these words to every doctor who encouraged the move. The tripping incident had bolstered my confidence. Bob hadn't fallen on *my* watch!

≈≈

On day sixteen, I flung the French doors open and came into the room, heavy-footed, plopping down a little too hard on Bob's bed. His eyes fluttered open.

"Dammit, Bob, I just got off the phone with your sister," I began.

"Hmm, yeah ..." Bob attempted an answer.

"I am so sick of her-you gotta be positive-attitude. People shouldn't ask me how I'm doing if they don't want to hear the truth. I was just trying to tell her how hard this is," I lamented.

Bob made a noise of support (I like to believe) and promptly fell back asleep. I continued ranting, oblivious to the fact that I was talking to myself.

"I'm being realistic. Why does *realistic* have to be seen as *negative*? I am hopeful, damn it, nobody wants to see this thing work out more than me, trust me! But I'm living knee-deep in reality here," I finished with an exasperated grunt.

As I thrust my hands out in front of me, my eyes swept the room. The colorful cranes, still shoved in corners and on bookshelves, did little to mask the IV pole and the syringes on the desk. I stared at the light coming from the sitting area. It fell across the gash on Bob's forehead, giving it a sickly orange hue. The curtains were drawn, and the air around my gaunt, gray, sleeping husband seemed heavy with desperation.

I sat there quietly for a while, my mind drifting to my checklist of chores: vitals in another hour, meds in thirty minutes, tube flushing tonight.

Bob sat up quickly and headed to the bathroom, using the IV pole as a cane. He was dizzy and had diarrhea, a bad combination. To make matters worse, the nurse wanted a stool sample from him to check for a possible bacterial infection. I handed him the bedpan for collection.

"What more humiliation and degradation can they put me through?" Bob croaked.

I put my head in my hands. *Yup, reality.*

≈≈

At day twenty or twenty-one, we were pushing hard for discharge from the co-op. Bob's low blood pressure was keeping us there. He was clear of infection but couldn't get his blood pressure up or his appetite back. We had hoped to be back at the apartment by the time Henry came back, but it seemed as though Bob's blood pressure was not following our plan.

Henry arrived back in Omaha with his Aunt Kathy, his sky blue eyes wide, giving us the Henry Stare when I opened the door and found them standing stiffly in the hallway. My nine- month-pregnant belly blocked the doorway and I was still wearing the latex gloves and mask needed for the dressing change I had just performed on Bob's central line. Bob cautiously stood up from the chair, careful not to get lightheaded from the effort, pulled his shoulders back, and raised his bony face toward his son.

Henry, standing in that dimly lit hallway, looked older than his three years. His eyes were weighted by all the thoughts swirling in his head, his body guarded, ready for the next blow. Henry looked at us as if we were apparitions. It had only been three weeks, but a lifetime had passed since we last saw each other. We were surely different people now.

How could we come back together from these different lives we had been living and resume our life as a family? Were we still speaking the same language?

≈≈

On day twenty-two, Bob returned from the workout room and performed deep knee bends in the sitting room before I took his blood pressure. We had been told that a top number of 80 or above would get us discharged. Henry watched the scene from the hospital bed, quickly bored with putting the head of the bed up and down. Kathy and I were boxing up our belongings, putting all the cranes carefully in a bag.

We all watched anxiously as the blood pressure cuff tightened around Bob's arm and the digital numbers began to tick off: 40, 60, 75 ... 80! Finally, reluctantly, the medical team gave us our freedom. We were sent back to the apartment with Bob's still-low blood pressure, pages of instructions, a handful of prescriptions to fill, and a reminder to report any fever immediately to the nurse.

One of the best parts of Cooperative Care was that discharge planning had begun as soon as Bob started the procedure. My intimate involvement in Bob's care gave me the skills and confidence I needed for an easy transition to caring for him at home after his transplant. There should be less professional intervention required post discharge. "Should be" was the key phrase in that sentence.

≈≈

In the end, I was too confident and too trusting about Bob's insight, wanting to honor him and our independent natures. The first evening we all kicked a soccer ball around the parking lot of the apartment building. The second night Bob spiked a fever.

"Bob, I need to call the doctor," I said hesitantly, staring at my hands in my lap as we sat side by side on the edge of the bed. Bob's sister, Kathy, was in the living room, and Henry was asleep in the room next door.

"No, Renie, I'm fine. I just need some rest," he calmly convinced me.

"Please, drink this water, try to eat something," I pleaded.

Wanting to respect his independence and his wishes, I went against my better judgment. A downside to being a care partner was my difficulty realizing that Bob was not making the best decisions for himself. The core of our relationship, our self-reliance, was challenged.

Being the main decision maker proved too big a task for me. Later that night, I felt Bob rise from our bed and then heard him crash into the closet.

"Bob, are you OK?" I asked, my heart beating in my throat.

"Fine, just going to the bathroom," he answered, annoyed.

I sat straight up in bed. My hand flew to my chest to calm my racing heart. Then there was a sick, heavy thud in the bathroom. I ran to the door and began pounding on the door, yelling for Bob. I was able to squeeze the door open and saw his legs splayed out and his head between the toilet and the shower stall; he had passed out cold.

"Bob!" I screamed "Oh, my God, Bob, get up, wake up!" I heaved my body down next to him, attempting to lift him up as he slowly came to.

I heard a voice from behind me. "Don't lift him." Bob's sister, Kathy, had awakened at the commotion.

We got him up and to the couch, where I forced him to drink water. He promptly vomited it all over the parking lot as we walked out to the car. Driving through the dark empty streets towards the Lied Center, I felt deflated.

"I'm so sorry, Bob. I screwed up. I should have called the nurse last night. I knew I should have called the nurse." I berated myself, and my heart continued to beat loudly.

"No, Renie, I'm sorry," he said, sounding befuddled.

≈≈

Bob was admitted to the ICU until a bed became available on the transplant floor. The transplant team came to the ICU for the morning rounds, interrupting my reading of *The Da Vinci Code* aloud to Bob. I felt demoralized by all their sympathetic stares at the two of us, lying in the tall bed in the dark, sterile room. They stood there with their clipboards and their knowing looks. They had all been right; we weren't ready for discharge.

Once Bob was an inpatient, I had less responsibility and became obsessed with getting Bob to eat, as if eating would solve all our problems. Sitting next to Bob on the bed, I perused the menu as if it had come from a five-star restaurant. I tried to ignore the nurse taking Bob's blood pressure. She never even offered the number to me; I had to ask.

≈≈

On day twenty-five, my mother and I were heading back to Milwaukee because my due date was rapidly approaching, and Bob remained in the hospital. Leaving without Bob meant I had to turn over his care to my father and Bob's brother, Eugene. Meticulously I went over the dressing change procedure and his list of medications for when he was discharged. Eugene had a one-liner for everything and a long mustache to fit his funny guy persona. Both men put on a brave face and carefully watched my demonstrations, glancing at the written instructions nervously.

My mom and I drove out of the city, and my heart felt sharp-edged from the guilt of ignoring Bob's fever when it had first spiked. My limbs felt heavy from my longing for outcomes beyond my control. My head was a jumble of worry. Would Bob eat, when would he get out of the hospital, would he be home when I went into labor, would he be in remission, would he live? What strength would I draw upon to birth a baby?

Luckily, Bob was discharged from the hospital later that very day, just three long days after being admitted. The three of them were allowed to leave Omaha just three days after my mother and I arrived back in Milwaukee. The car, loaded with the bikes and the kitchen utensils, picked up speed as it neared our home in Milwaukee.

I was picking up Henry at day care when the men arrived. Bob met us, and we three walked hand-in-hand down the sidewalk past the stucco duplexes and brick bungalows toward home. When we entered our back yard on that sunny, bright fall day, the air had an elated energy similar to that of an auditorium during a graduation ceremony, filled with a sweet collective sigh of relief. I heard no whispers among the coneflowers and the tangle of blue and purple cosmos.

The secret was giving me a bit of a reprieve.

The worst, we thought, was over.

Chapter Four

Dark Days

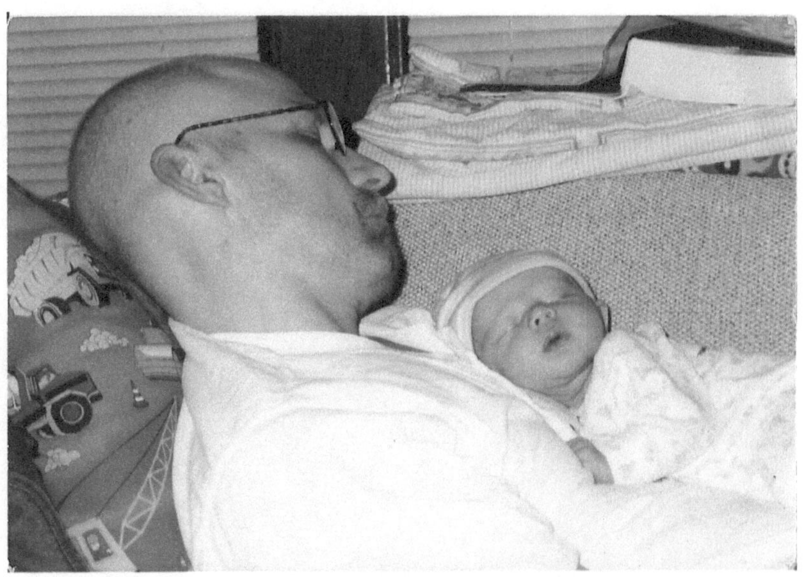

It is better to break one's heart
than do nothing with it.
Margaret Kennedy

"It's a boy!" The doctor made the announcement as he rushed to cut the umbilical cord that was wrapped around Arthur's neck.

And there was the cry, the newborn wail of a healthy baby.

And there went my heart, plummeting directly to my now-empty belly. The ominous feeling surrounding me separated me from the other people in the room. I was becoming increasingly irritated by these forewarnings. I wanted this moment to be pure light, without the darkness that waited at its edges, threatening to seep through.

I had had a premonition about this very moment long before, although I didn't recognize it as a premonition until just then. I hadn't thought about that dream in many years.

Bob and I were living in Portland, married and happily childless. One night I had the most vivid dream.

In my dream, Bob and I were in a hospital room, and there was light streaming in from the windows. We had just had a baby boy. Bob was beaming, looking down at his son. I watched them from the bed.

"You see, Renie, I told you everything would be OK. He's beautiful. We can do this," Bob gushed.

Joy radiated from him. His energy disturbed the dust particles floating in the stream of sunlight.

Looking at the two of them, I felt so peaceful and happy and calm.

The scene shifted, and I saw myself sitting on the hospital bed. I was smiling at the boys. The sunlight was now coming from a skylight above my bed. I was blanketed in the light coming from the heavens. I looked for the window on the wall. It was still there, but the blind was pulled down. I noticed the bright line of light that framed its curled edges, the bright sun trying to sneak its way around the curled blind.

When I awoke, a very peaceful feeling lingered.

Later that day, on the way to Mount Hood to go cross-country skiing, I told Bob about the dream.

"Maybe we could be parents, Bob. You looked so happy and confident. Maybe I would feel as peaceful with a baby as I did in the dream," I commented wistfully.

That afternoon was our first conversation about the possibility of having children. Three years later we had Henry. Three years after that, we found ourselves in a hospital room with light streaming in from the windows as Bob beamed at his son.

≈≈

The gust of wind that blew through the room and whispered to me went unnoticed by everyone else, enthralled as they were with the beautiful new life in the room. Bob's gaze didn't leave Arthur as the nurse cleaned him up and swaddled him before she brought him back over to me. Our friend Sarah and our doula (birth coach), Sarah, were watching from a distance.

Our doula hadn't been as essential this time around. Henry had come like an arrow released from the bow, anxious to make his appearance in the world. Bob and I hardly had time to be a team. Arthur came right on his due date and needed some persuading, as if he knew what he was getting himself into once out of the safety of the womb.

Outwardly and logically, I was happy he was a boy. I wanted a brother for Henry and I thought it would be easier to have two of the same sex. But I also had a theory of a soul replacing a soul, so the fact that we just had a boy, by that logic, did not bode well for Bob.

I had no rational cause to feel this way. Bob's progress had been going according to plan since we returned from Nebraska. Bob was back at work and had recovered amazingly well from the grueling stem cell transplant. He was in good spirits, cooking and riding his bike, engaged in activities. He hadn't been writing in his journal much at all.

Bob had been right, as usual. Back when he was first in the hospital and I was first pregnant, I had wanted to "get rid of it", even having a friend inquire about an abortion. The two of us lay on the hospital bed together one morning between tests. My red reindeer pajamas and the shamrock blanket I brought from home gave the bland hospital room a splash of color.

Bob had strongly discouraged me from making the appointment. "Renie, it's going to be Halloween then, and I'm going to be fine, and we're going to wish we were having this baby together."

Arthur was born during that brief window after returning from Nebraska when we thought Bob was well. His bald head shone in the glare of the hospital lights as he jabbed his fist in my back, and I hugged the birthing ball so hard I thought it might burst. After all those weeks in Nebraska when I had been the caregiver, now it was Bob's turn.

Trying to put Nebraska behind me, I was cautiously optimistic as the birth approached. I felt strong and full of energy, as after completing a difficult hike or a long, hilly bike ride. I figured that I had just successfully lived through the hardest trial I would ever have to suffer in my life.

I was counting down to our hundred-day follow-up appointment in Nebraska. Christmas would be day one hundred. Arthur was born on day forty-five. We had been waiting for so long to hear the word "remission". I was so looking forward to returning to the transplant center and hearing that word.

Remission—what a beautiful word.

I remember wanting the Denver Broncos to win the Super Bowl when I was about ten or twelve. I wanted that feeling of excitement and celebration and elation that I would see on the faces of the fans in the other towns, the winning cities. I actually got on my knees in front of a picture of Jesus that hung at the foot of our stairs and prayed for the Broncos to win.

Ridiculous, I know! It was just a game, right? Why would Jesus care? I had no control over the outcome of the Super Bowl, just as I had no control over the outcome of Bob's remission now. But I wanted that word. I craved it as a child craves love from an abusive parent. We had been beaten up, and now I just wanted one little word, a tiny show of affection; that didn't seem too much to ask.

I wondered how much one person could ask for knowing that I had used Arthur as a bargaining chip with the fates. I wanted Bob to be healthy. Secretly I hoped for a colicky baby or even a disabled baby ... if I could just have Bob healthy and alive and with me. I could handle anything if I could handle it with Bob.

But here he was: Arthur McGoldrick Wellenstein, born October 31, 2003, at 3:38 in the afternoon, and he was perfect.

And he was easy.

≈≈

Thanksgiving came quickly, and there was an energy shift in the house. The air became heavy like it does before a summer storm, the house grew darker, and we all slowed down and grew wary. We braced ourselves for the first burst of wind.

My parents came for the holiday. On the surface, the event was picture-perfect. A beautiful meal, a beautiful new baby, and our beautiful family and friends gathered around the extended table. In actuality, our lives were beginning to spiral down the way they had the year before, the fall and winter before Bob was diagnosed.

Bob had begun to withdraw and journal more, signs I wanted to ignore, but everyone in that house could see them. People watched his every move, trying to interpret every comment or twitch. For me, there was a spotlight on his shoulder. My eyes were drawn to that shoulder like iron filings to a magnet. I couldn't look away if I tried.

Thanksgiving afternoon I descended the stairs and turned the corner into the kitchen. I carried Arthur, who was in a pleasant nursing coma, milk bubbles forming on his lips. I found myself poised on the square landing, unable to move, startled by the sight of my dad and Bob as they scoured the turkey for enough scraps for soup.

It wasn't the sight of them there, heads bent over the carcass, veggies lined up ready to slice, that troubled me; it was the voice. The secret spoke again, and it sounded urgent.

"*Remember this moment.*" Starting at the base of my ribcage, the message circled around my head and shot down to my feet, cementing me to the stairs.

Bob left the room so abruptly that I was sure he must have heard it too.

"When will you go back to Nebraska?" my dad asked once Bob had gone. His eyes remained on the soup he was stirring, which now bubbled on the stove.

I shrugged my shoulders in response, still unable to move.

"Bob won't answer me when I ask him. I think he's nervous," I attempted lamely to explain, training my eyes on the carrots and celery floating and bobbing in the pot. A hint of the savory aroma that filled the kitchen tickled my nose.

My dad simply nodded. He felt the shift too. My charade was unconvincing.

≈≈

My parents went back to Colorado, and the four of us walked to the park near our house. Some leaves hung on the trees tenaciously, breaking up the bright blue sky with their dull yellow and rust. Bob and I were seated on a bench at the band shell, watching Henry run around. I had Arthur in the sling. Sitting on those benches always made me think about being in labor with Henry. I had been on one of those benches right then, hearing a jazz concert, unaware of what was underway.

Gazing down at Arthur's long lashes, I thought about the women who envied both of our boys and their long eyelashes. The lashes covered deep blue eyes that both Bob and I could take credit for. Stroking his blonde wisps, I remarked on the difference between the boys' hair.

"Remember, with Henry, how we joked that we should stop at the barber on the way home from the hospital?" I asked randomly.

If I just kept talking, then Bob couldn't talk. He couldn't tell me anything bad, such as why he didn't want to call Nebraska and make our follow-up appointment. Nor could he tell me why he was retreating to his inner world, why he was on the computer for hours each day, why he was journaling more, or what he was thinking about.

Please, Bob, just don't talk.

Then he talked. "Renie, I'm not in remission."

"FUCK!" I replied, just as plainly. I whipped my head up from Arthur's contented, sleeping face and glared at Bob as if he had just slapped me across the face.

"Shit, shit, shit! God damn it, Bob," I yelled at him. I think I might have hit him if I hadn't been holding Arthur.

"Renie, don't worry. I'm going to be fine. I'm still going to beat this thing," he responded, unruffled by my outburst.

"How? What else can we do? We've done everything, Bob. We went to Nebraska, for God's sake," I drew out *Nebraska* slowly, deliberately, a breath between each syllable, just in case he had forgotten about the trip. "All that crap you went through, for nothing. We have done everything," I screeched.

I was crying, again, resuming my familiar fetal position, bent over Arthur with my head in my hands. My hands pounded my head as if I could knock the words that Bob was telling me out and send them far away from here, where I couldn't hear them anymore.

"We haven't done everything. We're just now on the right track with all the holistic alternatives. I'm going to be OK." Bob said this as if he really believed it.

I wanted to believe it too. I always believed what Bob said to me; he was usually right. I wanted him to be right. I wanted to feel his hope, but all I felt was dread and fear. There was nothing else to do.

What else could we do? How could I be here? My mind raced.

Here we sat, holding our infant son, watching our three-year-old roam around on the stage on this glorious late fall day. A casual observer might have thought we looked like a picture-perfect family. Norman Rockwell could have painted our picture at that moment.

Upon further observation, would the picture have told the real story? I felt like that picture of the old/young woman that you study in school to learn about perspective. If you concentrate on the nose, you see the old lady. Look at the eyelashes, though, and you see the young lady. If someone looked at my arms, they would see a loving mom cradling her son close to her. If they looked at my hands, they would see a terrified woman gripping her son in an attempt to keep from spinning off her axis.

The wind was no longer swirling or whispering to me. It was a gale that whipped through me and left me stunned in its wake. Bob was talking; he continued to talk, but I couldn't hear what he was saying; he seemed so far away.

All I could hear were the voices in my head. *I am going to be a widow, a widow. What are we going to do? How will it end? How will I raise these boys without Bob?*

"Are you sure? How do you know? Have you spoken to the doctor?" I babbled these desperate, stupid questions, not even looking up at Bob.

He was sure. A person knows when cancer has returned.

≈≈

Bob's journal entry
December 5, 2003

The cancer in my shoulder has come back. I started to feel it about a week before Thanksgiving Day. I was pretty sure of what it was. It is so goddamn frustrating that after everything we have done, it just keeps creeping back.

I told Irene this past weekend. That was pretty hard to do. I got a PET/CT scan this past Wednesday and we are just waiting for the results from that. Even though I am certain it is back I think it is going to be disheartening to get official confirmation.

I feel in my heart I can beat this thing. Sometimes my heart sags and I feel hopeless but I bounce back and I renew my commitment to reverse this process going on in my body. I think we have allowed conventional medicine to run its course but I still believe that the nutritional, herbal, psychological and spiritual avenues I have been pursuing will pay off. The pain in my shoulder makes it difficult at times to remain optimistic. Yesterday, I felt unbalanced and frustrated and overwhelmed.

Cancer is really a son of a bitch, but it is not invincible.

≈≈

"I'm going to be a widow, can you believe it?" I told my sister Kathy over the phone, trying to desensitize myself to the word. My eyes were fixed on Arthur, who sprawled on his animal print blanket in the middle of the living room. My poor sister had innocently called to check in and see how Thanksgiving had gone.

"Oh, Irene, I don't know what to say … maybe not. You might get the results back, and he might be fine, and you guys can open a bottle of wine and celebrate," Kathy said weakly. She couldn't have believed what she was saying.

"I can't drink wine. I'm nursing," I said, martyred.

Hanging up the phone, I stared out the window at the bleak, gray day. A car drove down the street, my neighbor was hanging Christmas lights on his patio, and there were other people going about their days. Shaking my head, I swallowed what felt like a softball against my larynx. I was too afraid to start crying now, for

I might never stop. Shivering, I stood up to grab the baby and hold him next to me and try to absorb the warmth of new life—"Arthur therapy", Jeanne called it.

≈≈

Bob and I picked up the phone simultaneously, anticipating the call. Dr. Pierce was calling with the results from Bob's PET scan. Bob listened in the kitchen while I paced around the computer room. She was sorry to tell us there was a "hot spot" in his shoulder, indicating the cancer was back. The rest of the conversation was just white noise. My mind sprinted in another direction.

We met in the kitchen after hanging up. Bob leaned against the stove, watching as I milled about the kitchen while rearranging the silverware, afraid to look at him or utter a sound. If I didn't mention the phone call, it could not be confirmed; maybe I had simply misunderstood. When I finally stopped and looked in his eyes, they were quiet, almost confident. He wrapped his arms around me, and I felt my frayed nerves ease.

The second we parted, the current of anxiety returned. I felt my head nodding as if I understood as Bob summarized what the doctor had said on the phone. "Wait and see … talked to the doctor in Nebraska … stay positive."

"What are we supposed to do now? What's the plan?" I asked slowly. I meant right that minute, that night. I could not imagine what our next move was supposed to be or formulate a plan for the next twelve hours. I could not remember the last time I had nursed Arthur. I wasn't sure if the boys were both asleep right now or if they were even in the house. They might have been at their aunts' place, for all I knew at that point.

"We have to wait," Bob started to say.

"Wait? I can't wait any more!" I yelled at Bob as if he should have been able to find the cure for cancer right there in our kitchen.

It's over echoed through the kitchen, rattling my thin composure. I glanced around the kitchen, trying to locate the source of those words. Bob appeared not to hear them. He was still talking about diet and some new drug trial going on in Nebraska. His lips continued to move, but I pushed the mute button in my brain, only listening to that nervy voice that flustered me with its predictions.

"I think we should sell the house," I blurted out in the middle of Bob's talk about something he had read about peach pits. I suddenly felt very alone in that big house, and Bob's presence already felt less secure somehow.

"Renie, I don't want … I feel defeated when you say that, like you're writing me off." Bob spoke with a twinge of anger that I was not familiar with.

"This is not me being defeatist, Bob, this is me being realistic. This is me reprioritizing. If you were cured tomorrow, I would still want to sell this house. It's too much. I want to downsize. I need to simplify. I don't want to spend all of our time with this house. I want to go on bike rides and hike and go camping." I wanted these things so desperately.

≈≈

Bob's journal entry
December 9, 2003

Yesterday Dr. Pierce called and told us that the PET scan showed activity in my right scapula. I was not really shaken by the news since I already had no doubt that something was going on. And yesterday was a good day. I was feeling very optimistic. Irene was hit pretty hard by the news since she probably held out some hope that the news would be good. The upside for me was that the only activity was in my shoulder and that the CAT scan showed nothing. Dr. V. wants to get me into a clinical trial for a new MAB.

Irene responded by saying she wanted to sell the house. I know she is terrified by the idea of losing me but this reaction made me angry. I took it as a sign of her throwing in the towel. Selling the house was one of the first things that came to my mind after we met with Dr. A and we felt like all hope was lost.

There are times when I feel remarkably confident that I can turn this thing around and there are times when I feel like crawling into a ball and letting whatever is going to happen, happen.

I'm afraid to tell people this latest news because I don't want anyone to think my situation is hopeless. Cancer is not unstoppable and my body is remarkably strong. I have many resources at my disposal that I have yet to tap into.

≈≈

"Good God, Jeanne, I look like I have had a rough year. We can't use this picture! This picture is horrible. We can't send it to people. Look at us!" I lamented. If this Christmas picture went out to all our friends and family, then there would be no denying that we were a family in its demise.

The two of us were looking at our holiday photo, just taken by Jim, and I was comparing it to the one from the year before, also taken by Jim. Last year's was a gorgeous black and white taken before we knew Bob was sick, before we knew I was pregnant, before everything fell apart. That black and white picture had earned twelve thousand dollars for the Leukemia & Lymphoma Society when "Team Bob" used it in an appeal letter for a team my family organized for their Light the Night walk in Fort Worth, Texas.

"Well, it's a picture of a family," Jeanne responded in her pragmatic, upbeat voice, handing the current picture back to me.

This is not my family, I thought. I didn't recognize this group of people with their forced smiles and distant looks.

≈≈

The final notes of "Silent Night" hummed through the church. The smell of wax burning was strong as everyone blew out their candles and the lights came on. Kathy bowed humbly to the cheering crowd and acknowledged the children for their efforts, another Christmas concert over. I looked forward to this Wellenstein tradition every year, watching Kathy at work with her students, seeing the kids each year as they progressed through the Catholic grade school. I found the performance a lovely way to kick off the season.

We all stood up and began to collect our coats, scarves, and gloves. I scrutinized Bob as he situated Arthur in his infant car seat. He buckled him in and carefully, tenderly tucked the fleece blanket around Arthur. Could anyone tell? Did anyone else see the worry lines around his mouth, the distant look in his eyes as he went about his fatherly duties?

We hadn't told his family the bad news yet.

Helping Henry with all his cold weather gear, I saw Kathy unbuckle Arthur and pick him up. Her creased chestnut eyes only saw Arthur. Her smile was so genuine as she cradled him in her arms. Jealousy jabbed me with a force that took my breath away.

Was anyone noticing how strained our smiles were?

≈≈

Bob and Henry came home with the Christmas tree one bright afternoon, filling the house with the fresh scent of pine. The strong, spicy smell did little to clear the stagnant air that hung in the house like the dense haze of a bar after closing.

Henry was into cutting and taping anything he could get his hands on, so he and I made a star out of aluminum foil while Bob fussed with the lights on the tree. The two of us made the saddest, most pathetic and lopsided star you would ever see. Henry was so proud to place it at the top of the tree. Bob and I hung back, not wanting to infect Henry's exuberance with our gloom.

Torturing myself with thoughts of last year's Christmas, I remembered how Bob and I had lain on the couch under the blinking red and green lights and stared at the stockings hung over the fireplace, wondering how anyone could be as lucky as we were. Blissfully unaware of the maverick cells running amok in Bob's body, we had talked about having another baby. I had explained to Bob that we had to have another baby because I saw four stockings hanging up on the mantel next Christmas.

Well, the four stockings hung there now, just as I predicted, and all I could do was cry. Tears seeped out of my eyes, inundated from the flood of emotions bearing down around them. Through this waterlog, I watched Henry stretch from his perch on the ladder, completely focused on getting that shiny, lopsided star on the very top branch, and I could not conjure a picture of four stockings hanging on the mantel next year, no matter how I tried.

≈≈

Bob's journal entry
December 28, 2003

Arthur is not sleeping well tonight and that makes two of us. I took 10 mg of oxycodone and that usually gives me a weird alertness. The pain in my shoulder is enough to keep me awake at night so this leaves me between a rock and a hard place. The pain is not bad during the day unless I'm doing a lot of walking or just standing up. I had a massage the day after Christmas and it was incredible. The therapist Rita is also a cancer survivor so we talked about that afterwards.

This crazy ass cancer is really something else. I've kicked this thing so hard and so many times that I almost have to respect it for coming back for more. Rita said something about how she came to view cancer cells as being weak and confused and that she believed they could be returned to their normal state or if not that then just sloughed off. That is what I would like to do with this giant mound on my shoulder. I would like to slough it off.

Tomorrow we go to meet with Dr. Pierce. She had been looking over treatment options for me. In a way, I feel like we are in a better position than when I was initially diagnosed. We're educated and we are for all practical purposes done with the chemo regimens. I know my body, mind and spirit can fight this thing. I need a little help with the shoulder area but I feel and believe that everything else is under control.

≈≈

Staring at the yellow smudge on Bob's pillowcase, I sat hunched over Arthur while he slept, snuggled between breast and pillow. Everything in our house was turning yellow—the countertops, the sheets, Bob's clothes, his hair.

Bob had read about turmeric and its anti-inflammatory properties. It could shrink tumors, the information stated. So he dutifully concocted a turmeric poultice, and I dutifully rubbed it on his shoulder three times a day. And now everything these poultices touched was turning a muddy yellow.

Clinking things around in the kitchen, I could hear Bob efficiently mixing up the reddish yellow paste. Reluctantly I rose from the big chair to lay Arthur in his crib so I could go downstairs and get the chore over with.

Of all the alternative methods Bob was trying, this one made me the queasiest. We ate enough flax seed to last a lifetime. We bought a ten-pound bag of carrots, some ginger root, and a juicer. Bob chewed on peach pits and ate Brazil nuts. He drank a mushroom tincture. He agreed to esoteric healing and to an evaluation by an EPFX (electro-physiological feedback xrroid) machine. He stood on one foot and turned in a clockwise circle and repeated, "My immune system is strong and capable." He meditated and listened to inspirational tapes.

But the turmeric poultice seemed like just one more task I had to perform before I could go to sleep. Bob was receiving some experimental treatment and had another PIC line inserted, so we were back to flushing tubing and changing dressings. I fobbed off whatever work I could on the visiting nurse who came to administer the treatment.

Steeling myself for each application, I would smear the poultice on the increasing mass that lay between his spine and his right scapula. Bob asked me to massage oil into the skin that stretched, taut and itchy, to accommodate the tumor's increasing size. Holding my breath, I took a Sharpie and outlined the tumor, trying to keep track of its growth.

Given the choice, I would have rather drunk a gallon of the mushroom tincture than touch that tumor. It was this entity, all its own, a relative who had overstayed all welcome. I was afraid to give it any negative energy, lest it feed on that. I tried to befriend the tumor and talk kindly, explaining that while we learned a lot from its visit and did appreciate that, it was now time to leave.

≈≈

Bob's journal entry
December 31, 2003

Shoulder is really starting to bother me. I've been surprised up to now, given how large the tumor is, how much function I had retained in my arm. Now I'm starting to see some real limitation. I can still drink and eat and hand things to people with relatively little discomfort but anything beyond that is becoming painful. My shoulder is huge and disturbing to look at. I wonder if this is what caused the hunchback's hump.

≈≈

One night, as I spread the yellowish paste over the mass, I could feel heat coming from the tumor. It wasn't just warm like a sunburn; it was hot like a stove. My hand reflexively moved away from it. I tried shifting my attention to Bob's hair, which was coming back in. It was darker, wavy, with a strange, smooth texture, as if not sure it wanted to stay on his head.

My eyes shifted abruptly back to the tumor as if drawn by that magnet. The mass seemed to pulse under my hand like the rumble of an active volcano. There was energy, a simmering anger to this entity that I did not understand. We had tried to make friends with it and nicely asked it to leave, but the tumor seemed to react with vengeance, as if it were an oppressed people refusing to be kept down a minute longer. This entity seemed to be staging a coup, erupting from Bob's body because it couldn't come out any other way.

What was it? Why all the anger? Where was it coming from? Bob had such a calm, peaceful manner. He did not seem angry at all.

Believing in the mind-body connection, I tried to put the pieces together. Why would a healthy, active young man in the prime of his life be hit with this aggressive cancer?

Bob's silent struggle with depression was the only explanation that made sense to me.

Bob used his journaling to exorcise his demons, confess his doubts, share his observations, write poetry, and clear his head. It was the same way he used his love of nature. Both of these were quiet, meditative activities, turning his anger inward.

Bob struggled with self-doubt throughout his life. He lacked social confidence. This strain manifested itself with his introspection, his contemplation, his reticent nature. There was no anger anymore, not outwardly. He kept that to himself.

This fact was his greatest gift and his largest fault. For people who were able to experience his calm and gentle way of interaction, his temperament was a great comfort. Bob was level-headed, well-read, and cerebral. He was a very thoughtful, understated conversationalist.

However, his temperament was also his greatest fault. Keeping all this negative energy to himself, he was never able to be free of any of it. Eventually he was unable to tap into that emotion at all. He just buried it and stuffed it so far within himself that it finally started a grassroots rebellion.

Standing in the kitchen, staring at this angry mass on Bob's shoulder with paste that looked like brown mustard dripping from it, remembering the events of Bob's childhood and our life together, it became so clear to me. It was impossible to separate his illness, born in the blood of his body, from the fact that he had spent the better part of his life containing his pain in one compartment of his psyche—curtained off from the rest of his emotions and only accessed in very controlled circumstances. His journal and his therapist saw bits of it. I saw only the smallest hints.

Anger and bitterness were simply not emotions that Bob used in his interactions with the world outside. And I now believed they might be playing a part in his death.

≈≈

There was a lot of crying in cars. What is it about a dark car that makes it feel like a confessional? Jeanne and I would return from a movie, and she would just keep driving while I talked and we both cried. Driving home from work, I would sometimes find myself cruising around any random neighborhood, taking advantage of the only time I had alone, returning home after I had finished crying.

One evening I had a particularly difficult time getting the car to drive in the right direction. I was reliving a conversation with my boss, Beth, earlier that day. Beth had known me since I was twenty-two. She was my first boss out of college and was a mix of mentor, friend, and mother. Earlier that day she had been giving me the pep talk that so many others had given me before. I mean the one about all the other people she knew who had been living for years with lymphoma and how we might too.

I was dumbfounded by people's lack of understanding about our dire situation. I felt as if I spoke *ad nauseam* about the whole thing, but few seemed to understand that Bob was not in remission, had never been in remission, and would never be in remission. I suppose that no one who had not witnessed the rapidity of the progression could imagine its speed.

"Nothing is working, Beth. Bob and I are not growing old together," I stated firmly. She sat in my officemate's chair across from me. Her long, strong face remained calm, but the wrinkles around her hazel eyes crinkled and gave her sympathy away. I leaned toward her to emphasize my point, stopping short of tapping her on the head. "We already aren't Bob and Irene anymore. We haven't been Bob and Irene for a while now." Averting my eyes from her pained look, I tried not to think of what the words meant as they escaped my mouth.

When the car finally found its way home, I found Bob and Henry with their arms in a bowl of flour, pizza fixings lined up on the counter, and an odd mix of garlic and pineapple in the air. The periodic table of the vegetables framed in red above the counter reflected the overhead light and Arthur watched them serenely from his bouncy seat in front of the dishwasher. Bob looked up at me with a carefree look in his eyes before noticing my telltale red and swollen eyes.

"What's wrong?" he asked sincerely, as if the PIC line weren't dangling from his arm as he kneaded the dough.

Everything. You won't be here to make pizza with Henry in a few months, and I have no idea how to work the Kitchen Aid, for starters.

"Some days are harder than others," I answered out loud.

Bob nodded casually and returned to his rhythmic kneading. Stealing a chunk of the cool pineapple as I passed by, I bent to pick up Arthur and walked towards the couch, leaving the two of them to their creation.

Well, maybe we were still Irene and Bob, at least for tonight.

≈≈

Bob's journal entry
January 16, 2004

> I love the relaxation angle of this tape but I have a
> difficult time with the visualization aspect-especially
> the healing place stuff. I am not entirely happy with
> my healing place. It is a cottage in a forest near a
> river and I don't know if it is the whole *Deliverance*
> similarity or what but it doesn't seem exactly right.
> Something seems to spread out about it and there
> is no focal point. I don't know what my other ideas

would be for a healing place—a cave somewhere in the mountains or a more religiously inspired place like a chapel. I think I need a place less remote than my riverside retreat. I need a place where people would be found.

≈≈

My family began to rotate in, only letting a few weeks go by in between visits, each person offering her or his own unique style of support. My sister, Colleen, was the spa sister and took me for a hot stone massage. The warm stones gliding over my limbs on that cold January evening penetrated the tension encapsulating me. Walking out of that room in a steamy aromatic fog, I marveled at the flexibility of my body. The room would need to be cleared of all the anxiety that spilled out on that table.

Afterwards I basked in the relaxation room in my big fluffy robe while waiting for my sister. The room was warm, the light was low, and I curled up with my peanuts and water and tried to remember the last time I felt so nurtured and peaceful. Wincing a bit, I recalled Bob's attempt at romance just the other night.

He had called me at work, expressing body image issues and the desire for us to be alone, even securing child care with the aunts for the night. Bob even asked if I had been given the go-ahead from the doctor following Arthur's birth. I didn't have the heart to tell him I had been cleared for quite a while now.

When I walked into the bedroom later that evening, I tried not to weep. The candles Bob had lit and the pink blanket he draped across the bed gave the room a smoky look. He was so earnest about his desires, and it suddenly felt like our first time.

We slowly lay down on the bed, careful to avoid any position that would bother his shoulder. Bob reached for a condom out of the drawer.

"We sure won't need that!" I quipped. If the chemo hadn't killed off everything, I was sure all the painkillers he was on would make it impossible for him to finish the job.

"I just want to be sure," he said quietly, his expression so sincere.

I willed myself to wrap my arms around him with no hesitation as he removed the fleece shirt I had been wearing all winter. I was careful not to touch any rubber tubing from his PIC line or put my hands directly on the tumor. Closing my eyes, I was able to enjoy the pleasure of our skin touching; his arms around me were reassuring. Looking beyond the medicated cloud, I saw only trust and love and desire. We kissed tenderly, and his lips felt a bit rough and dry from the medication.

"I love you, Renie," he whispered hoarsely into my ear. A trembling in my chest brought back long-forgotten memories, as a whiff of a scent will bring you back to that magical vacation. Desire and love flooded me without warning, like a flash flood on parched earth.

Bob's head suddenly felt heavy on my shoulder, and I realized he had passed out, his breath warm on my skin. The candles continued to flicker, and silent tears streamed down my face. The unused condom mocked me from the bed.

The candles were out when I woke later, seeing the moon full and bright outside the window. I stretched my hand out for Bob. A chill ran through me when I found only familiar, cold, damp sheets where he had been sweating earlier. I sat up and saw him sitting in the big chair, head bowed, dozing.

≈≈

Bob's journal entry
January 29, 2004

I had a scare yesterday. I've been having night sweats and the night before last I woke up at one point completely drenched in sweat. Around 5:45 AM I got a call from my dispatcher who said all she had for me were middle schools so I chose John Muir which I've had some experience with. The nice thing was they didn't start until 8:10 so I crawled back into bed. I figured I would get back up around 6:30 but I ended up staying in bed until a little after 7:00 AM. When I did get up I felt incredibly dizzy and weak and I thought I might throw up. I wasn't sure I was going to be able to go to work, and a whole host of darker thoughts started in motion. The dizziness passed after awhile but everything I needed to do to get ready seemed to require a Herculean effort. When I got to school I got out of the car and walked to the building and up a couple flights of stairs. This left me completely out of breath and exhausted. I felt better as the day progressed and by the time I got home my energy had returned. I felt nervous about the prospect of another morning like this and worried about the effects of another infusion of the ganite given these events.

This morning was much better though. I took two oxycodone before going to bed and Irene gave me a foot and head massage. I slept pretty well and when I woke up and got out of bed I didn't experience any of the dizziness or fatigue of the previous morning.

≈≈

The "big chair", as it was affectionately called, was in the guest room and served many purposes in our household. Bob had proudly brought it home from a secondhand shop one day. He loved a bargain. The Wellensteins were masters at finding a bargain and fixing things. Nothing would be thrown out or replaced if it might one day be fixed with a little duct tape or bungee cord.

When Bob and I were first dating, we were strolling down the city street I lived on, pointing out the buildings in need of repair, discussing what we would do to them to restore their splendor if given the chance. Then Bob suddenly disappeared inside an apartment dumpster. He sprung back up with a Kirby vacuum in his hand and a smile like a kid's grin in a candy store. Bob proceeded to roll that vacuum down the street beside us.

"Why are you taking that?" I whispered loudly, with more than a note of disgust, feeling suddenly very conspicuous.

"Because I'm a Wellenstein," he told me proudly, as if no other reason were necessary.

That vacuum brought us years of good service, and so did the big chair. It was oversized and fluffy and had an ottoman; it was big enough for us to snuggle up in on a rainy afternoon and read the paper. After Henry was born, it became the nursing chair and then the bedtime reading chair. Lastly, when it became too painful for Bob to sleep lying down, the big chair became his bed.

From the guest bed where I was propped up and nursing Arthur, I watched Bob, sitting in the big chair, knees over one arm and his head resting on the other. He was reading "If You Give a Pig a Pancake" to Henry. Bob kept nodding off in mid-page turn. His head would sag forward, but his thumb kept working the page, wearing a hole right through the words "so she'll want to take a bath.". After a minute his head would bounce back up, and Bob would continue reading in a husky voice.

Henry sat and waited each time, studying the pages in front of him, fingering his fleece pajamas with the tools print. The motion was much like Bob's way of fingering the pages of the book. I thought Henry might wear a hole right through a hammer or a wrench. After a time Henry began to produce big sighs and not-so-gentle nudges to encourage Bob to remain alert.

"Mommy, can you finish reading the story? Daddy's too sick to read," he finally asked, losing patience.

These words woke Bob, and he looked toward me, trapped on the bed with Arthur happily sucking. Bob rose and slowly but purposefully walked out of the room, his shoulders hunched with the effort of stifling the great sobs emerging from someplace primal. I watched him, unable to move, helpless to comfort him. Henry looked at me expectantly, waiting for his book to be finished.

"Come on over next to us on the bed, Babe," I said, patting the bed beside me, listening to the stairs creaking under Bob's weight as he headed towards the living room. In that moment I not only understood the word *heartbreak*, I felt it happen. If I looked hard enough, I thought I might see half my heart follow Bob down the stairs while the other half remained rooted with me where my boys had me surrounded.

The thought of Bob downstairs, alone, with the realization that he was dying creeping up on him, drove me to distraction. Getting the boys to bed became a series of tasks performed by reflex; my thoughts were only with Bob. I could only hope he felt them.

When I was finally able to join Bob on the couch, he was looking straight ahead in contemplation. The red of his flannel shirt was the only color I could see in the dark living room, and the only light in the room came from the street lamps. I could have used some of his practical advice on what I should do or say in this situation. When our legs touched, it was as if he had an electric current running through his body.

"I'm scared, Renie," he said, head down as if making a confession.

"I know, Bob. I know. I'm so sorry I can't be there for you the way you need. I watch you, and I wonder what it is like to see your son and know you won't ever see him play Little League. But I don't ask you because I can't handle the answer. I am so worried about remaining upright for the boys that I can't begin to feel what you must be feeling, or I might dissolve into a puddle right here on the floor." I attempted to explain my position and absolve myself of guilt for not being the ultimate caregiver and nurturer, for needing him too much during his time of need.

Bob didn't say anything; he didn't have to, I could feel his acceptance wrap around me like that old comfortable blanket. He just lay his head on my shoulder and let me hold him while his whole body shook with sobs.

Bob's journal entry
February 6, 2004

I didn't sleep much last night. Not sure why. Henry and Arthur went to bed great and I was in bed by ten. Sleeping is not uncomfortable but I do have to be picky about position and I am tethered to this pump. That wasn't it though. I just felt alert, not really restless.

Tonight Irene and I are going out to dinner with Sarah & Garrett to 3 Bros. We are leaving all of our assorted children with Kathy & Jane. They're going to have their hands full.

This is turning into a long day I wasn't prepared to sit on my hands all day. I'm bored and eager to get out of here. I'm looking forward to tonight, hanging out with S&G. Enjoying good food, good atmosphere, maybe a beer.

I have snow to shovel when I get home. I'm tired of shoveling snow. We have so much there's nowhere to put it. I have to push almost all the snow in the driveway down to the front of the yard. And our snow blower doesn't work.

≈≈

The two of us watched as Dr. Pierce closed the door behind her, giving us some "time alone", as she had put it. We sat there like two lost kids at a baseball game, hands in our laps, squinting under the fluorescent light, waiting for our parents to come save us.

Only no one was coming to save us.

"Go home and enjoy your family, Bob," she had told him. We all know what *that* means.

"Henry does have his last tumbling class on Saturday," I had responded weakly. I was not looking forward to taking him there, alone yet again, while Bob sat at the hospital, alone, getting a blood transfusion. But if he did come to tumbling, it would just highlight the fact of how many things Bob wouldn't be doing with Henry in the future.

"Any more chemo, and I worry that you could die of a stroke in your sleep," Dr. Pierce had explained matter-of-factly. Strongly discouraging Bob from further treatment, Dr. Pierce had also mentioned hospice care, predicting that with no more treatment, he would be dead in three weeks.

Three weeks?

The idea of death by stroke during sleep sounded wonderful to me. The idea that the end could be that near and that painless brought sweet relief percolating through my veins. It sure as hell beat the projection that the doctor had just provided for us in response to my continued pestering to know how this cancer would play out. In excruciating detail, she had explained how the tumor would get larger and larger and constrict his lungs and heart. The damn thing protruded so much on his back already that I was afraid it might break through his skin and explode. Yes, a stroke in his sleep sounded lovely.

"Renie, the last ten years … you have been the best thing …." Bob stammered, grabbing me and pulling me toward him, his words hot on my collarbone.

"I know, Bob … don't …" I stopped abruptly and just held onto him as if we had just been shoved off a plane and he held the only parachute. My mind was racing with all kinds of inappropriate thoughts: *don't do this, Bob, don't say anything, not now, not here, I can't handle it, my eyes are still swollen from yesterday, I can't walk out into that office with everyone looking at us, knowing.*

That afternoon Bob chose further treatment, believing that he just had to shrink the tumor enough to get some laser procedure he had read about that would blast the tumor. He wanted this even after Dr. Pierce had explained that the tumor was too big; she even explained that she didn't want to schedule another PET scan because she didn't want Bob to see the actual size of the tumor. That sight would be too demoralizing. "A football" was the description I remember.

What I wanted to say to him was: "Bob, it's over, please, no more treatment. I can't go to any more doctor appointments. Just the thought of walking into this office with all these people and their sympathetic looks turns my stomach. I just want this over. All the ugliness needs to go away. I'm drowning here."

What I did say was, "You have to do what you want, Bob, what you feel is right."

We walked out of the exam room and then in opposite directions. Bob headed straight to the treatment room, and I went straight to the elevator, trying to keep my eyes down and not look at anyone. I caught a glimpse of the blue fake leather recliners lined up along the windows in the treatment room, an IV pole paired up with each one, as if on display as a matched set. I tasted the sting of bile as it rose in my throat.

Finding myself at Sarah's house, I expressed to her all the things I couldn't say to Bob while her eight-week-old daughter, Clara, cried for her in the living room. Sarah sat next to me on their bed, her arm around my shoulder, and tried to keep her own emotions in check. It felt so scandalous to admit I wanted Bob gone, to hear my voice speak the unspeakable.

"You just want all the ickiness to go away," Sarah said quietly, understanding perfectly my dilemma.

"He's already gone. Bob's already gone," I kept repeating, my head in my hand, in defeat.

Later, driving us home after his chemo, we discussed signing up for palliative care. Palliative care is just like hospice care except that the patient can still be receiving treatment, as I explained to Bob. So we would have access to a social worker and nurses to call if or when something happened.

"Why do we need that, Renie?" Bob asked. "What can they do for us?"

"Bob, you don't want to go back into the hospital, right?" When he nodded, I continued. "I need someone to call if something happens." Visions of him falling down the stairs danced in my head. "You have to do this for me, Bob. This is for me," I said emphatically, feeling the tide shift.

It wasn't all about Bob anymore.

As soon as we returned home, Bob took off on a bike ride. With the phone clutched to my ear, I watched him ride down the street with Henry secured in the trailer behind him, dirty mounds of snow still visible along the road in the vanishing light.

"He could be gone in three weeks, she said. He's on a bike ride right now, for goodness sake." I attempted to explain the contradictory life I seemed to be living to my sister, Anne.

"Wow, you hear all this talk about quality of life. I guess that *is* quality of life. I just thought when it got to this point, you would hear *six months* or something," she trailed off.

"It's better this way. If it's going to be over, it's better to be quick. I don't know how I can watch this, I couldn't handle six months," I croaked, feeling the secret fill the room with its unending babble of prophecies and anxieties.

The late winter light came through the long windows and cast eerie shadows across the living room. I hugged myself, trying to shake off my cold, wet fear.

≈≈

Jane and I were talking on the phone while I traced Henry's perfect red lips in the picture that sat on my desk. There seemed to be a lot of talking on the phone at work and not a lot of working. My officemate respectfully pretended she didn't hear a word of my conversations. Jane was trying to talk me out of keeping Bob at home with hospice care, telling me that she and Kathy could find a place for him to go.

"You have to think of yourself. You can't do all of this. You don't want the boys to see this." She tried to convince me.

But that was exactly what I did want. Given our situation, I strongly felt that the only way Henry had a chance of understanding any of this was by witnessing the progression of Bob's death. That, also, was what Bob wanted. At that point I had no idea how I would manage, but I knew I would, since I had to.

"Jane, I love him." My voice was heavy with tears that I was trying to keep from falling.

"I know you do," she responded with equal emotion in her voice.

"He would do the same for me." I had no doubt about that.

As soon as Jane and I hung up, my phone rang again. This time it was Nicole, a friend whose husband had the successful bone marrow transplant in Nebraska, just checking in. Filling her in on the details of our latest doctor appointment, I braced myself for the uplifting, encouraging comment that would probably follow. "You are strong", or "You will be OK, it is so great you have those boys", or the uncomfortable silence that usually followed the word "hospice".

"Oh, Irene, you're in for some dark days," she told me.

Hearing the stark truth spoken was utter relief. The tears were sprung free. I felt them on my cheeks and tasted the salt on my lips, so cleansing. It was true that I was strong and that kids are resilient and that I would get through all of this somehow.

But I was in for some dark days.

≈≈

Sitting in the big chair with Arthur, who was curled around me and blowing milk bubbles, I listened to Bob and Henry's voices coming from the bathroom across the landing. The two of them had been showering together since Henry was old enough to stand up safely. It was a task I had gladly handed over to Bob, who could instruct him on proper hygiene on boy parts.

I heard Bob's gentle guidance over the water: "Now it's time for the soap …"

And then Henry's high-pitched boy voice: "Daddy, why do you have to wrap up your straw with that plastic stuff before you get in the shower?"

I marveled at Bob's patience and focus with the instructions and explanations he was providing for Henry, as if he had nothing else on his mind. For that moment the activity in the house was so normal: nursing, showering, parental instruction, nurturing. I wished they could stay in that shower forever. The minute they were out, I knew that I would have to change the dressing on the PIC line for Bob, and soon after that he would be groggy from the pain medication.

≈≈

Bob insisted on another PET/CT scan even after Dr. Pierce had done her best to explain that further scanning was pointless and would only upset him. I could not bring myself to drive him to that appointment. The mere thought of it made the contents of my stomach curdle. Jane agreed to take Bob.

Blinking back tears, I watched Henry run after Jane's car as I proceeded to secure the car seat in our Subaru. Flinging in the diaper bag, neatly packed with breast milk and diapers, I heaved my briefcase onto the passenger seat and called for Henry to get in the car and buckle up.

"Bye, Daddy!! Bye-bye, Daddy," he joyfully sang out, waving his hands at the car as it disappeared down the street.

≈≈

Bob's journal entry
February 17, '04

I am so fucking bored and aimless it's incredible. These last few days of subbing have been characterized by clock-watching and overwhelming ennui. I yearn for Friday. This is a 3 day weekend coming up so it will be wonderful.

I want to beat this cancer thing but what if I did beat it? I don't need to change anything radically but I do need to start making changes. I like the idea of getting involved in Yoga and imagery work because of the relief these things have offered me during this time. Rock climbing, chess, speaking Italian, all these things I want to do.

I feel so useless at this job. I yearn to utilize some skill or ability. I sit here knowing nothing, doing nothing, just a pair of eyes. I just want to get back on track. I want to finish my teaching certificate, explore some other career options, move on.

The other night Jeanne and Jim were over. I still feel weird about how disconnected I felt. I felt lost there too, adrift. I worry that I have become increasingly withdrawn in the last couple of months. I don't think I ever really acknowledged how devastating the recurrence was after the transplant. I feel like now I am balancing on the thinnest of tightropes and the slightest disturbance will cause me injury.

≈≈

Hustling out of the bathroom to get back to Arthur, whom I had left lying in the middle of the bed in the guest room, I almost ran right into Bob. He stood teetering at the top of the stairs, one hand on the banister and one foot suspended on its way to the first step. Frozen in place, I stood stranded on the landing halfway between the bathroom and the bedroom. Out of the corner of my eye I could see Arthur scooting his way towards the edge of the bed.

Staring at Bob, framed by the dark orange tulips of the stained glass window at the bottom of the stairs, I envisioned him tumbling down the stairs and crashing into the window, the shards of yellow, red, and orange sparkling as he lay in a heap at the bottom. That was not how I wanted him to die at home, not with panic and chaos and possible blood. I hesitated only a moment between my son rolling off the bed toward the radiator and my husband tumbling down the stairs. Gently taking Bob by the shoulders, I guided him to the big chair while Arthur gracefully landed on the floor with a thud.

His gaze unfocused, Bob allowed me to manipulate him into the chair as if he were a demented man of ninety. After assuring myself that he was secure, I picked Arthur up to assess any damage; he wasn't even crying. He just looked up at me quizzically, as if to say; "Where were you?"

Holding Arthur tightly to my chest, I recalled my conversation last night with Jeanne. I had asked her to watch Bob for me while I went to give a massage. Driving to work earlier the same morning, it had occurred to me that I could no longer trust Bob with the boys alone. Bob had been so confused and shuffling while he attempted to pack the boys up for day care. The week before, Bob had run into the side of the house with Henry in the car on an excursion to

Simma's Bakery for cinnamon rolls. That accident should have been my first clue.

Returning home from the massage, I found Jeanne and Bob on the couch, a single lamp turned on, in the same positions as when I had left them. Bob was opening a CD player and closing it again methodically.

Leaving him on the couch with the CD player, we spoke in hushed tones in the kitchen. Jeanne told me that at one point in the evening, Bob had accused Jeanne and me of trying to "trick him". It was no wonder he felt tricked—all the whispered conversations that ended abruptly the minute he walked into the room.

Jeanne was trying to soften her no-nonsense message: it was time to call in my people. I was afraid to call people in too soon. Not knowing how long the end would be, I didn't want to put people out for too long. Several coworkers had signed up for shifts starting later in the week, I explained.

Jeanne looked at me, her eyes awash with unshed tears. "Irene, I think it's time. What are you waiting for?"

"I'm waiting for things to get really bad."

She just shrugged her shoulders and gestured slightly with her head toward the living room. There Bob sat on the couch, his head now sagging and the CD player splayed across his lap.

≈≈

Later that same evening, after Jeanne had left, after I checked in on the boys and got myself ready for bed, Bob wandered up to the guest room and sat on the edge of the bed. I sat down next to him, hoping he couldn't read my mind. The light from the landing made a triangle on the carpet. I watched him in dejected silence as he fiddled with a Ziploc baggie. Bob had substituted a plastic baggie for the CD player.

He turned abruptly to me. "I know you think I'm crazy," he stated defensively, looking perplexed and hurt, as if falsely accused of a crime.

"No I don't, Bob," I tried to reassure him and myself. However, he was acting like many of the folks with dementia who spent the day at my workplace. "I'm just scared that something's going to happen and I won't be able to handle it." This was a genuine statement, and my arms went around him as if I were comforting a child.

He straightened up and shook off my embrace, turning his gaunt, gray face toward me. He took my hand and spoke with the reassuring tone that I had come to count on throughout our relationship.

"Renie, don't worry. You will." Our eyes held each other's, and in that instant it was as if the last year hadn't happened and he and I were discussing a bike ride that I was worried about or a parenting issue I had been insecure about. "Renie, don't worry," he always said to me, aggravatingly sure of himself.

Then the instant was over and he drifted away again, back to working on the baggie. I sat for a moment and hoped Bob would return and reassure me again, but Bob was gone. Leaving him on the bed like this, just a shell, I slowly crept down the stairs. I folded up at the bottom, my head between my knees. The house felt so big, and I felt so insignificant and alone even though there were four humans living within these walls. The lights from the kitchen felt like a spotlight on me, as if an audience out there in the dark waited for me to perform. I had no idea of my next line.

Only I did know what my next line was. I had to start making the phone calls, and once I started them, there would be no turning back. I was about to embark on a one-way trip. The troops would mobilize and the house would fill up, but I would still feel empty, and the house would still have the bleakness of an empty theater. Unwillingly, my hand went to the phone hanging on the wall; it seemed to dial without my permission.

"Anne," I said on a deep shaky intake, "it's time."

≈≈

March 2004
Want List

Rock gym membership
Motorcycle

Learn a martial art
Learn to sail
Write more letters

≈ ≈

Mourning March

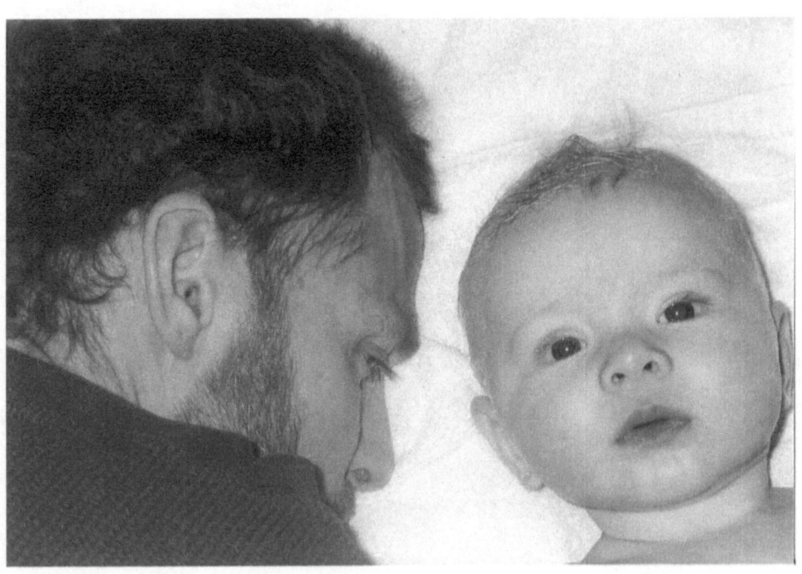

You and I got a piece of an infinite thing.
From the reaches of the universe,
I'll be callin' callin' your name.
Peter Himmelman, *Measure*

≋

The soft morning light drifted through the window and subdued the blue walls. Arthur lay on Henry's bed; his hair was damp and his cheeks were still pink from his bath in the sink. Arthur kicked and squirmed, his arms reaching out towards me as I warmed the oil in my hands, preparing for his massage. His head moved with the effort it took to talk to me in four-month-old language, "oooh, ooooh, ahh, ah, haaaaaaaa," all the while looking so earnest about what he was telling me.

Kneeling beside the bed, I leaned towards Arthur and took hold of one restless leg, making firm long strokes towards his toes, slowly inhaling the lavender from the oil.

"Don't worry so much, don't hurry so much …" I sang to him absently.

Willy Porter had been one of the six CDs in our player for the past two days. I hadn't thought to change the music.

"Go easy on yourself, it's what I'd do … I'd go easy on myself, if I were you …" I even swayed my shoulders a bit and tried to add some harmony. Arthur's eyes were round and wide and satisfied. They reflected none of the worry that had taken up permanent residence in my own. He was focused singularly on me, and for a moment I felt his uncomplicated gaze surround me and offer me comfort as surely as if he were giving me a big hug with those tiny, warm, and sweetly oiled arms.

Bob silently glided into the room as if he were part spirit already. His energy only added to the tranquil force filling the room. Bob was glassy-eyed and slightly unsteady, as if he'd had one too many glasses of wine. He wandered over and knelt down next to me beside the bed. Without a word, he bent forward and laid his head next to Arthur's and slowly closed his eyes. Bob remained that way, asleep, while I finished the massage and dressed Arthur.

Leaving the room, I could feel the shift in energy hit me as if there were an electric fence around the doorway. Turning back I saw Bob, unchanged, bent forward over the bed as if in prayer. I was jealous of the peaceful energy that immersed him; it covered the room like a fine warm mist floating up from a waterfall.

I resisted the urge to jump back in the room and drown in its tranquility. I had planning to do for the arrival of my people. I had called in the troops, circled the wagons, and later that day, the first of them would arrive.

≈≈

With Bob still asleep upstairs and Henry still at day care and my sister not arriving for a few hours, I decided to give Arthur his first serving of "real" food. Arthur was almost five months old, and I couldn't put it off much longer. No time like the present.

After I prepared the soft boiled egg and mixed the yolk with a little water, I carried Arthur, in his bouncy seat, to the middle of the living room. Sitting in front of him with my legs stretched to the sides, I thought for a second that I should go wake up Bob and bring him down here for this milestone. Then I remembered his lack of enthusiasm when Arthur had rolled over by himself for the first time just the other day and how deflating that had been. I tried hard not to think about when Bob and I had given Henry his first egg, the laughter we shared as Henry clasped his little lips around the spoon and drooled yellow ooze down his chin.

I flipped on the TV to drown out the silence of this moment and proceeded with the spoon toward Arthur's eager mouth.

≈≈

March ?, 2004: Bob's Last Journal Entry

Affirmations

I am healthy and my immune system is strong and capable.

≈≈

Kneeling on the couch with Bob slumped in his La-Z-Boy next to me, I watched Anne get out of the taxi cab and furtively look around the neighborhood. Rolling her suitcase past the street lamp, she was briefly illuminated before boldly walking up the porch stairs. I half-expected to hear her start singing "I Have Confidence" from *The Sound of Music* as she stood before the front door, poised to knock.

Arriving on Thursday night, Anne was the first.

Next, on Friday, came Mike from Portland.

The moment when I finally understood Mike's offer to come and help meant he would serve as an oncology nurse, was a turning point in this final act.

During our phone conversation, I had repeatedly assured Mike that we would be fine, explaining that my sister was coming the next day and that there were also Bob's family members and folks from work who had offered to do shifts. Honestly, I had no idea what to expect or what we were really going to have to do or how we were really going to do it. We just had to be fine—that was all I knew.

After hanging up the phone, I put Arthur on my hip and walked from the boys' room into the guest room next door. There Bob sat on the floor, leaning against the ottoman of the big chair with his legs stretched out in front of him like a big rag doll. The bright afternoon sun shone across his lap, where a plate with an orange cut in sections lay. The sweet, tangy smell made my nose tingle. Bob stared at the contents of that plate as if he had never laid eyes on an orange before and had no idea how to proceed with the task of eating it.

I eased Arthur and myself down to the stiff carpeting and leaned against the bed facing Bob. The nurse found us in that position when she arrived to check in. When she expressed great concern regarding my ability to handle the situation, I gave her the party line—we were fine.

"Don't worry," I assured the nice lady with the very concerned furrow across her brow, telling her that I was soon to be surrounded by support. We had lots of help. They just weren't here now.

"Bob will eventually get himself up and wander into another part of the house," I told her. "He isn't stuck here forever." I thought that fact would make her feel better.

Nodding soberly, she appeared unconvinced and left quickly to go back to the office and report to other staff her concerns. The three of us remained as we were. Watching Bob sprawled there, I pondered the issue of whether he should stay here while I went to pick up Henry from day care or if I would feel better with him on the first floor of the house. Last week he had been drawn often to the basement, where he had always worked on his bikes, and I didn't want him to get stuck down there.

As I weighed the pros and cons of each option, my most recent conversations played through my brain like a skipping record, stuck on the word "fine". Were we really fine? I felt maxed out with my nursing skills. One more dressing change or pain patch to keep track of, another doctor appointment or middle-of-the-night nursing, and I might run screaming out the back door.

All the care-giving details of my life had me feeling disassociated from my body. The heavy and worried portion separated and hovered nearby so that the rest of my body could move about its various responsibilities, unshackled but not unburdened. That troubled portion remained close and loomed large.

Suddenly a flash of understanding interrupted my thoughts, and I realized what Mike meant when he said he could help. Running toward the phone before the thought left me, I dialed the Portland exchange.

"Do you mean that you could come out here and care for Bob, like TAKE CARE of him?" I sputtered the second Mike picked up the phone, feeling a bit like Helen Keller might have felt with her hand under the running water.

Mike arrived two days later, in the middle of the paperwork extravaganza required to switch from palliative care to hospice care. Holding Arthur in one arm and signing the papers with the other, I listened as Mike spoke with the visiting nurse about pain medication. After hearing the word "mucosa" mentioned several times, I gratefully took off the nursing cap that had been weighing me down and handed it over to Mike. I could now be Bob's wife. I felt lighter already.

The last to arrive were Mark and Amy, having moved back to Minneapolis from Portland several years earlier. When the two of them entered the house, our care-giving team was complete.

≈≈

Once the team was in place, we all fell into our roles naturally, and the atmosphere became a magical mixture of hospice and frat house. Anne was the house manager, Mike was the nurse, Mark was the advocate for both patient and family, Amy was the rock-solid volunteer, Bob was the noncompliant patient, and I was the stunned family member. There were photo albums open on the dining room table, good music on the CD player, the smell of generic casserole being prepared in the kitchen, a hospital bed in front of the fireplace, *The Lion King* on the TV, and the doorbell and phone ringing nonstop.

The darkness of the last few months was blown wide open with the entrance of these four people; daylight streamed in from every window and door. Before our helpers arrived, everything seemed to happen at night when it was dark and cold and lonely. Now we were living during the day again, with the rest of the world, with the sun.

Initially Bob held court in the big chair that Anne and I had hauled down the stairs for him the first night she arrived. Friends and family came to visit and say their good-byes or drop off food. Some spoke to Bob in serious tones, while some simply reminisced about a recent trip as if they planned on seeing him again soon.

I wondered what Bob comprehended of all this activity. Did he know what it meant when Anne had entered the house? We had spoken together about calling her in if things got bad. Did he know things had gotten bad?

If Bob understood what all these visitors signified, he gave nothing away. There were no Hallmark card moments with me or anyone, no moments of great insight or acceptance. His attention span was short, and it was not long before the conversation took place around rather than with him, and his gaze drifted. I sincerely hoped he would die in that chair, simply drift away in the middle of a conversation.

≈≈

The progression was rapid in those last few days, and Bob's mental state was as unpredictable as the weather. At times he was serene, and at other times became very agitated. On Saturday Mike and Mark decided they were going to give Bob a bath, using the newly acquired shower chair. This meant that they had to get Bob from the first floor to the second floor. Bob was still independently mobile at this point, but only when he decided to move. He could remain in one spot, lost in thought, for hours at a time. Anne woke up Saturday morning and found him stuck in the bedroom on the third floor.

Later on Saturday evening, hiding in the shadows of the foyer, I watched silently as Mike and Mark tried to coax Bob up the stairs. Standing halfway up, they encouraged him as if he were a toddler just learning to climb stairs. Bob went up the first few steps, Frankenstein-like, and then abruptly changed his mind and turned around. The men instinctively reached out to Bob, who responded to their touch by grabbing onto the banister and gripping it with both hands and the strength of a man being taken to the guillotine. With Bob as the rope, a tug-of-war began.

Eventually Bob was led into the bathroom. It was not long before I heard him scream, followed by much commotion and scrambling in the bathroom. Apparently Bob had not taken kindly to the cold water being turned on him in the shower.

This can't be good. Leaning against the wall I sunk to my knees feeling as if I should pray for forgiveness. The high ceilings and cool darkness of the foyer mixed with the red and yellow of the stained glass window next to me did have me feeling a bit churchy.

≈≈

Amy seemed to appear out of nowhere and entered the kitchen. She was coming from the living room, where she had been visiting Bob, who was now immobile in the hospital bed. It was Sunday.

"This is so fucked up," she said to no one, wiping tears from her eyes.

I stared at Amy over the counter. There I had perched on a bar stool while watching Anne check on the latest gift of food, which she had warming in the oven; it smelled like tuna. Now Amy is not the kind of gal to use that kind of language, preferring something along the lines of "fiddlesticks". Also, I had specifically mentioned to Amy, when we spoke on the phone, that the use of that particular word was out when my sister Anne was in the house.

Of course, I had told Amy that when I was repeatedly dropping the "f-bomb" during our conversation.

"I'm sorry—I just keep saying "fuck", but my sister will be at the house tomorrow, and I won't be able to say it anymore, you just don't swear in front of Anne." I offered as an apology to the silence at the other end of the line. Telling Amy that Bob was dying had been so hard, making the whole thing so real somehow.

After Amy's comment in the kitchen, she and I froze with our hands to our mouths, feeling like busted school kids. We both chanced a glance at Anne.

"I'm sorry," Amy shrugged feebly.

"Not at all, I think on this occasion it is quite appropriate," Anne answered without skipping a beat.

There ought to be a name for laughter mixed with tears.

≈≈

"Mommy, why does Daddy's breathing sound like that?" Henry asked, turning his serious face from Bob's and walking the short distance from the hospital bed to the dining room table.

Amy and I looked up from the pictures from a hike we had all done on Mount St. Helens eight years ago. I immediately looked to her for an explanation of death rattles for my three-and-a-half-year-old.

It was still Sunday.

≈≈

"Irene!" Jane called up the stairs. "Come on down here." It was about 9:00 PM then, and still Sunday.

My heartbeat accelerated when I heard my name. Anne and I were hiding on the third floor, trying to avoid seeing Bob's mom standing next to him by the bed. I claimed that they needed their privacy, but the truth was that I didn't think I could handle seeing a mother looking down at her dying son.

Jane and Kathy had just arrived with Bob's mom and three of her sisters, fresh from their brother-in-law's funeral in Minneapolis. Reluctantly I came back downstairs just in time to hear one of Bob's aunt's lean toward another and say; "Isn't there something they could do for him in the hospital?"

I observed these sturdy, elderly women from the safety of the stairs. You could tell they were sisters by their broad shoulders and the way they all inhabited the space around the bed, as if they had been sharing space all of their lives.

They don't get it. They don't see what I see. They only see what isn't there. I was disheartened.

I saw the mantel above the hospital bed and the family pictures on display up there, our smiling, familiar faces. I saw the big chair with its big red flowers and our old gray couch right next to it, so dull that we had to fold my grandma's pink afghan across the back for color. I saw my care team blending into different corners of the room, respecting the family but not willing to leave their posts. I knew the boys were tucked in their beds just one floor up. I could hear "Breathe" playing for the hundredth time on the CD player. The room had a glow as if there were a fire crackling nearby.

We were home.

I wanted Bob's family to see what I saw, how perfect everything was.

"You did the right thing," Jane whispered to me, still on the stairs. "This is just wonderful."

I exhaled breath I didn't know I was holding.

≈≈

My eyes shot open in the dark. Henry was asleep next to me. The numbers on the clock were a smear of red. Was that a four?

Attempting to orient myself, I tried to think of the day. Monday, maybe?

Where was Bob?

Something lodged in my chest like a boulder. Lifting my head off the pillow, I couldn't seem to get a deep breath, and something was swirling around the room. I felt a breeze and thought the window might be open.

"*He's gone.*" I felt the words bang back and forth in my head.

Henry stirred and coughed—a wet, throaty one like a bullfrog.

"He will need honey lemon tea," I thought vaguely.

Then I felt a hand on my shoulder and turned my head away from Henry to see Mike bent over the bed, arm outstretched. Like a sleepwalker, I rose out of bed immediately and headed for the stairs, hesitating as I turned the corner at the bottom.

There was Bob, lying quietly in the hospital bed. He hadn't moved from there in almost two days. Images of the last few days cascaded through my head like a waterfall, landing with a crash in my stomach, the spray dispersing through my body and making my fingers tingle.

Where was the raspy, wet sound of Bob's breathing? I thought as I lurched towards the bed.

Standing over Bob, I first looked down at his face; he looked comfortable, peaceful. My eyes moved to his chest, looking for movement. I kept looking for the up-and-down motion that I had been watching for since he had been in the bed. Still leaning over

Bob, I turned my head toward Mike. I could barely see him in the dark as he stood motionless in the middle of the living room.

"Is he gone?" I asked. Mike's head barely moved in an up-and-down motion. I sensed movement to my left—Mark, hovering in the dining room.

I looked back at Bob's face, which was still peaceful. No pain lines around his eyes or across his forehead. No struggle for breath or understanding.

Where is the relief that's supposed to rain down on me at this moment? All I feel is regret. I wasn't with him in the end. All the weeks in Nebraska being his nurse, the months following Nebraska that we had spent trying every crazy alternative therapy he came up with, the flushing of tubes and dressing changes. These last three days spent massaging his feet. And then I wasn't there with him when he died. I was in bed.

Henry came creeping down the stairs in the midst of my mental tirade.

Shit, not yet, I'm not ready.

But there he was, in the living room, all three and a half feet of him, giving me the Henry Stare. Standing in the half-light in his too-small blue fleece PJs, the pants reaching just below his knees. Moving to the couch, I took him on my lap, facing me.

"Henry," I said. That was all I could say. Nothing else came out. He waited, eyes moving to his dad and back to me.

I looked beyond Henry to Mark, still hanging at the edge of the dining room, the dawn starting to peek around the blinds behind him.

I looked at him imploringly. "I have to tell him, don't I?" I hoped he might give me some way out of this moment.

Mark's head moved slightly up and down, just as Mike's had earlier. *Damn both of you and your subtle head nods.*

"Henry," I looked back at him now, focused on my task. "Daddy ... he ... died, he's dead," I told him bluntly, telling myself at the same time. Henry nodded calmly and blinked those long lashes, just like his dad's.

We hugged awkwardly, and I glanced towards the stairs. There was Anne, halfway down with Arthur squawking a bit in her arms. She looked at me apologetically.

Man, this is outrageous. I held Henry's stiff body a bit too tightly and looked out over his boney shoulder. *I just told Henry his dad's dead two minutes ago, I just looked into Bob's dead face. Now I'm supposed to breast-feed?*

"He's gone," I said to Anne, stating the obvious. She moved her head up and down slightly. *Did the three of them talk about this?* I could imagine them plotting their subtle head bobs and telling one another to keep Irene guessing.

I motioned for Anne to bring me the baby as I moved Henry off my lap and reached for the nursing pillow.

≈≈

The group of us waited around the dining room table for the undertakers to arrive. I counted the nurse from the hospice, myself, Anne, Mark, and Mike. Henry and Arthur were somewhere nearby. I am not sure when Jeanne arrived. She had been on her way to work when I called her with the news. The blinds were now up and the light from the sun started to drift in and warm the room as the morning progressed. I held on with both hands to my now-empty mug, staring at the few foam bubbles left at the bottom from my morning chai.

Mark had been the chai maker since his arrival two days earlier. Bob had made my chai for me in the mornings up until about five days ago. I allowed myself just one chai per day, an extravagance I continued since developing the habit back in Portland. From the sounds that had been coming from the kitchen, I would need a new espresso machine. The familiar *skrrrrr* of the machine sounded labored and went on for way too long. Then, when Mark would hand me the mug, the chai was lukewarm and barely frothed. But I drank it, grateful for the warm and comforting cinnamon smell.

The drink was comforting but also set off in me a dull sense of anxiety, a chain of thoughts. *Who will make me my chai now? I guess I'll have to learn to use the espresso machine. I will just give up drinking chai. Yup, I won't drink it anymore, the machine is about to break anyway, and I will never be able to go to the store and buy a new one, I don't do that stuff, I hate that stuff, Bob does that stuff ... did ...*

The undertakers arrived in the midst of my fretting and began their work to prepare Bob for the ride to the mortuary. Would we like to leave the room while they prepared the body, they asked. None of us budged.

"What are they doing to Daddy?" Henry asked me as the men worked sheepishly at their job of washing Bob's body, wrapping it in a big white sheet, and placing it in the black bag, ready to transfer onto the gurney and wheel it out of the house.

"Taking care of him," I explained, distracted, wondering what time it was and if I could start making my calls.

Mark stood up and reached for my mug. I looked at him dubiously, gripping the handle a bit tighter.

"Irene," he said, arm still outstretched, patiently waiting for me to hand over my mug, "I think it's a two-chai day."

≈≈

Anne came with me to the mortuary later that same day. Bob would be cremated, so I thought this meeting would be simple. There were still plenty of decisions to be made. For instance, I still had to pick clothes for him to wear because I would need to view him in the casket to assure that it was the right body. And I still had to pick a casket because he would have to be in one to be cremated—that, the morticians explained, was the law.

As I walked through the showroom, I was struck by the absurdity of this situation—picking out a casket to cremate your husband in must be in the fine print of the marriage handbook, the part you never read. There were some plain caskets and some ornate caskets, and there was quite a range of prices.

Then there was the cardboard casket.

"Bob would kill me if I wasted money on a casket," I said to Anne. I knew that for sure. There was to be no viewing. That was a clear wish of his as well, made during theoretical discussions of death on hikes and the like. So cardboard it was.

Anne and I stood in the doorway of the viewing room. The aisle leading to the casket seemed very long and had some kind of bluish or grayish carpet. The room was cold and dark and smelled sterile, too sterile. It reminded me of a formal living room in a house that doesn't get many visitors; it felt devoid of life.

There was Bob, at the end of the aisle, looking very small, laid out in his neon fishy pants made famous in Nebraska.

Bob is in a cardboard box, this is ludicrous, this is what jokes are made of. I suppressed the urge to laugh out loud. There is nothing that can prepare you for seeing your husband in a cardboard box. *I wish Bob were here, we would have gotten a good laugh out of the whole thing.*

≈≈

Back from the funeral home, I was now the one to hold court. Sitting cross-legged on the couch, I told the story for the hundredth time that day to my boss and a few other coworkers who had stopped by on their way home from work.

"It was just how I wanted it ... if he had to die, it was really perfect ... but I wasn't there ..."

Suddenly Henry appeared in the living room.

"When is Daddy getting home?" he inquired; this would have been the time Bob usually got home from work.

I felt all eyes on me, and my heart skipped a beat as I wondered how to deal with this situation as everyone listened.

"Henry, Daddy isn't coming home. He died," I told him. My tone tried to convey that we had been through this already and please don't make our guests uncomfortable.

"You said those men were taking care of him," he retorted, challenging me.

That WAS what I had said, I chastised myself.

I hemmed and hawed a bit before spitting out a more pointed version: "I meant they were taking care of his body. He won't be coming home again," I said, as if this statement might make the situation clearer for Henry. Then I threw in "ever" for good measure.

Henry just nodded and left the room, leaving the adults to ponder what had just transpired.

≈≈

Later that evening, after the boys were asleep and the doorbell stopped ringing, I became obsessed with ridding the house of anything that reminded me of cancer, attacking the stacks of paperwork on the dining room table with single-minded focus. Anne and Mike helped me make sure, in my purging, that I did not lose something of vital importance.

Having already lost Bob, I figured nothing else could matter all that much.

We made a pile of all the CT scans and PET scans and his doctor's notes, visualizing a bonfire and all of her neat block writing, organized like a spreadsheet on the page, turning to ash. Books on cancer that Bob had collected and information he had printed off the computer all went into the growing pile for the garbage.

Reaching in Bob's briefcase, the black mesh one he had been taking with him to his appointments and transfusions, I found all the items he had last touched. They included the book he had been dozing off over for the last few weeks, *Angle of Repose*, a pen, some printed information sheets on alternative treatments he had been ready to discuss with the doctor, and a pad of paper.

The pad of paper with the flowers on the front was not the usual spiral notebook Bob used for his journals, and I flipped it open to the first page.

"Dear Renie", I read in Bob's slanted print, a bit spindly-looking.

"Oh, my God," I screamed, dropping the notebook back into the briefcase as if it were a snake. Putting my hand to my chest, I tried to keep my heart from bursting through my ribcage.

"What is it?" Anne was immediately by my side and peering in the briefcase, afraid of finding something alive and coiled up inside there.

"It's a letter from Bob. I just can't handle it right now. I can't read it," I stammered, shocked by my reaction to seeing his handwriting, such a solid thing, proof that he was just right there. I kept staring at the briefcase as if Bob himself might come popping out next.

"It's ok," Anne told me calmly. "Just put it aside. You'll read it when you're ready." She made every reaction I had seem like the perfect one for the moment.

≈≈

A gorgeous white two-tiered cake stood before us on the counter, and the faint smell of lavender and lemon filled the kitchen. Anne, Sarah, Jeanne, and I were silent as we gazed at the creation. "Happy Birthday, Bob" was written in yellow and purple icing.

Sarah had ordered the cake for Bob's fortieth birthday, and today was the day, April 2, 2004, a Friday. He had just missed it.

Now what do we do? Should we sing? Should we eat it? Should we just stand here in a huddle around the counter and stare at it? Cry?

The sniffling and shuffling began, and finally someone asked, "Are we gonna cut into it or what?"

≈≈

By Saturday my four sisters, my parents, and my sister Teri's two children were all in town. I had to wait almost two weeks for the minister to get back in town for the memorial. This gave me plenty of time to plan the perfect memorial, complete with our friend Willy playing the guitar, and to book the nature center for the event.

The enforced wait also meant that there was a lot of time to entertain guests, since people started to arrive immediately following Bob's death. There was a lot of car washing and vacuuming going on to fill the time. Now that my care-giving team had been replaced by my family, the roles were a bit different but just as efficient.

Anne was still the house manager, but she now teamed up with Kathy, who was very good at following orders. My dad took on the role of taskmaster, my mom was in charge of paperwork, my sister Colleen was the activity coordinator, and Teri and her kids seemed to be in charge of child care. The two kids were very accommodating of Henry's strange ideas of play at that time. I remember the "Owie" game being very popular. What the rules or the point of it were, I am not sure. I continued in the role of stunned family member, good for nothing. I couldn't even tell them where the vacuum bags were when they asked.

Someone suggested a good, old-fashioned "McGoldrick dinner" one evening. So, after the necessary shopping and Thanksgiving-like cooking frenzy, we sat around my dining room table and passed the platter with chicken and Total-cereal crust clockwise. Steam rose from the mound of whipped potatoes, and the corn provided our only color on the table.

The average cacophony around a large dinner table was going on.

"Please pass the …"

"Did anyone see …?"

"Have you …?"

"Ahhhhhhhhhhhhhhhhhhhhhhhhhhhhhh!" Henry, seated next to me, shrieked, unprovoked, in the midst of it all.

Conversation halted as everyone turned to stare at him. Looking at Henry and his face while he screamed, I felt helpless and envious at the same time. If it had been socially appropriate, I would have loved to do the same at that moment. How freeing a primal moment like that would be!

≈≈

The days until the memorial passed in a blur of visitors, and food, and meetings, and even one afternoon of manicures planned by our activity director. The memorial finally arrived, and I stood on my front porch with four of my closest girlfriends, who had just arrived in town, and we watched as the last of my family drove down the street, the red taillights barely showing in the afternoon sun as they stopped at the corner and turned left towards the highway. They were surrendering my house to my friends and me for the next two nights, and the boys were with the aunts, who would be bringing them to the memorial service later that evening.

I waited only a few seconds before I turned to the group of women and pointed to them accusingly. "ok, who's got them? Who has the cigarettes?" I knew that one of these women, these girlfriends from my childhood, this eclectic group of women who had seen me through my formative years and closet-smoking years, would have thought ahead and would have them for me. It was our pattern, what we did when we saw each other. We were now adults and parents and environmentally aware and health-conscious, but whenever we were together, it was just us girls, someone had a pack, and we lived frivolously again for a few days.

The two of them who were not pregnant reached immediately toward their pockets and produced the contraband. So one hour before my husband's memorial service, I sat on my front porch and smoked like an addict fresh from rehab while rattling on about the pressure I felt to stay healthy for the boys and wondered if anyone had any perfume to cover the tobacco scent on my clothes.

≈≈

"I'm worried about Henry," I told my coworker and her husband, my eyes darting about the room trying to locate him amongst the mourners.

The nature center was filling up with clusters of people, some looking at the picture boards the aunts had put together, others idly stroking the snake and fox skins at the tactile station, some sitting in front of the fireplace looking out at the just-budding trees bending in the wind off the lake. The sounds of the chain gang from *O Brother, Where Art Thou* echoed in the room.

How does the widow handle herself in this circumstance? Is there a receiving line? Did I need to talk to everyone? Do I console the hysterical friend on the other side of the room, someone I don't really know?

There are dress rehearsals for weddings and weeks of classes for childbirth, but nothing for funerals. One is supposed to put together a party for a large group in just a few days and then act appropriately, but what *was* appropriate, especially since we weren't doing the traditional wake/viewing where the rules are better established?

"I'm just worried about Henry," I repeated to the tall couple before me.

"Kids are resilient," the husband responded.

Staring at him blankly, I thought for a moment that he hadn't understood what I had said, but then I realized he had understood me; we were just talking about two different timeframes. "No, I mean I'm worried about him *right now*. I am worried about him getting through the memorial with all the people and attention."

There was no way I could think past this memorial and worry about how Henry was going to *be*. I was literally living from moment to moment.

There is nothing like death to force you to live in the present.

Moments later Henry and I got stuck in a doorway on the way to our seat. His bulky winter coat felt coarse on my cheek as we got squeezed together in another group hug by well-meaning friends. I caught a glimpse of his painted lavender fingernails peeking out from the arm of his jacket. He had absolutely insisted on painting them after my sisters and I returned from the manicurist the day before.

"Don't you want to take your jacket off, sweetie? You'll be so warm." A couple of the well-meaning friends attempted to coax Henry out of his coat.

Henry responded with the Henry Stare and a subtle nod of the head, indicating that the jacket was staying on.

"Come on, dear, I can hang it up for you," the friends continued on their mission.

"NO," Henry responded, beginning to struggle against the hands reaching out toward his jacket.

"Don't hurry so much, don't worry so much." I could hear Willy starting to sing in the front of the room.

"He's fine, it's fine," I assured the couple; removing their hands from the collar of his jacket so I could pick him up. Turning blindly, I hurried up the aisle to the front of the room. There the urn sat, bookended by two bouquets of fuchsia and white wild flowers, Henry still perched on my hip.

≈≈

Henry remained glued to my hip throughout the service, mesmerized by the "man in the white robe as he talked about Daddy", eyes wide while Willy sang "Measure" by Peter Himmelman and "Watercolor Sunrise" by himself. He changed his focus to his aunt from Atlanta, sobbing next to us, while my dad spoke about Bob and our families. He remained undistracted by Mark's strong voice as he read his assigned poem.

But when I tried to get him to take his seat when I got up to speak, he was right back to the hip; he was not leaving my side. There we stood in front of the crowd, me in my butterfly sundress and Birkenstocks and Henry in his winter coat and painted fingernails. I attempted to share cohesively my thoughts on community and how I had learned that it was still alive and well.

Spotting Arthur in the crowd on my sister Anne's lap, his wispy blond hair all static and shiny in the sunlight, a smile on his round face, I lost my train of thought. I started recognizing others in the crowd: Mike, back in town from Portland; Margaret, on the aisle, brown eyes red and face blotchy; Bob's friends from work, standing in the back. A coworker of mine I hardly knew was there—so nice of her to come. I couldn't focus on any one face for too long for fear of absorbing any of their pain, for fear of feeling any of their pain, for fear of feeling anything at all.

I wanted to thank people individually but I began to feel a little bit like an actress at the Academy Awards. I was doing a rather good impression of a young widow, but I didn't want to forget to mention anyone by name. I thought I heard the guitar strings. Was Willy playing me off the stage?

"Thank you, all of you, I'm overwhelmed, we are so lucky," I stammered as I looked down at Henry, stoically looking out at the people. Kissing the top of his head, I repeated, "So lucky."

Lucky? How, exactly?

Yet that was the word that came to me. My husband was dead and I had two boys, one three and a half years old and one five months. Not my idea of luck, really, but I suppose I felt lucky to have all these people around me at that time, in that place.

≈≈

The day following the memorial, my family was dispersed throughout the living and dining room, surrounded by billows of torn newspaper. The living room was full of newspaper strewn about by Henry, who'd been ripping each section of the Sunday paper into long shreds. The piles spilled out into the foyer, like Christmas morning gone very wrong. I wished I could display my anger and confusion so tellingly throughout the house.

Everyone was waiting for the appropriate time to leave for the airport.

Sneaking out to the backyard, I sat in a folding chair and shielded my watering eyes from the bright sun, staring at the purple crocus starting to open up, the iris just poking through the dirt. I was so grateful that it was spring and there were signs of new life everywhere—longer days, a brighter sun.

Anne came out and sat down next to me.

No, not yet, don't leave me. Your husband will be fine without you. How will I function without you? Who will take care of things? Who will get the boys ready? I don't even know where the vacuum bags are, remember? I can't do this on my own, this is crazy. You need to move in.

I wasn't sure if these were voices screaming in my head or if I was saying any of this out loud. I desperately wanted Anne to stay. On the other hand, I couldn't wait to have my house back to myself, and I wanted to get the first night over with. I needed to get a day under my belt, then another. Was there any way to fast forward?

What I really wanted was to get the boys to bed and sit out on the porch in Bob's ugly old La-Z-Boy chair and smoke the remaining pack of cigarettes my friends had left for me. Was six PM too early to put them to bed? Everyone should be gone by then.

"I can come back whenever you need me," Anne was saying. "I was thinking mid-May I could come back."

I nodded, sniffing and wiping my eyes, staring at some weeds growing in a crack in the concrete of the driveway. I didn't want people to feel bad about leaving me or think I couldn't handle solitude. There would be plenty of time to fall apart once they all left, once I was alone.

≈≈

Even though there was no longer anyone camped out upstairs in my bedroom, I chose to sleep in the guest room for the duration of the time in that house. It just seemed safer, somehow, to have everyone on the same floor. That was what I told myself on that first night, anyway, when I crept out of the boys' room and stood alone on the landing, wondering which way to go. I had nothing to do suddenly, no one to worry about at the moment.

I woke up the next morning, not even aware that I had ever gone to sleep. Henry stared me in the face, asking for a smoothie, and Arthur whimpered from the next room to be nursed. I lay there for a minute while trying to put the pieces together. Why was I in that bed, in that room and alone? Then Henry insisted that he had to see my feet, and Arthur's whimpers turned to cries.

I forced my body to an upright position, got out of bed, and boldly walked down the stairs to the kitchen and faced the brand-new espresso machine; the one Garrett had brought over and carefully instructed me on. The blender stood there, empty and sinister. The thought of getting the yogurt and bananas and flaxseed oil out seemed an enormous task. I must remember to prepare the smoothies the night before, I reminded myself.

I placed Arthur in the bouncy seat, put an egg on to boil for him, and got the yogurt out of the fridge. I put the smoothie fixings in the blender as Henry arrived in the kitchen, dressed for the day. I turned to face the espresso machine.

The desire for a chai, something comforting and normal, forced me to face the unknown. Heck, if I figured it out, I might even allow myself two as a reward.

≈≈

We went to our first dinner, without Bob, with the aunts and Grandma.

Henry was edgy before we left our house. He was a jack-in-the-box, ready to spring, but not with a happy face. Sitting at the table next to him, I could feel him winding up, getting tighter and tighter each time I tried to settle him down. I felt wound up even tighter than he was, if that were possible. I was trying to put on a happy face for when I popped. Everyone was as polite as possible, ignoring Henry's unruly behavior and my unruly attempts at managing it.

Finally I grabbed him around the waist and took him from the table. My throat felt so clogged that I couldn't even explain where we were going. We went into a spare bedroom that had a futon. All but dropping him on the floor, I knelt down in front of the futon as if to pray. Raising both arms above me, I folded at the waist and slammed my fists down on the futon.

"I'm so mad," I yelled. "Ahhhhh, what am I going to do?"

Henry became mute immediately and watched in intrigued horror.

"Come on, Henry, hit the futon. Hit it as hard as you can. Go ahead and yell louder." I encouraged his hesitant first swing.

We beat that futon flat; we beat it until we were hoarse and weak. Then we returned to the dining room, where dessert was being served as if nothing were amiss, Arthur was still asleep in his bouncy seat.

The next day I went and bought Henry a punching bag to use at our house.

≈≈

Then came my first day back at work, and I was on my way to a meeting, trying not to make eye contact with anyone in the hallway for too long for fear that they might ask me how I was doing. Bob had been dead two weeks and one day, and I was afraid I might answer a little too honestly.

Despite my efforts at avoidance, I found myself face to face with a coworker.

"At least it's better than a divorce," she said, laying one hand on my arm.

Peering into her green-flecked eyes, I stood there, immobile. There was motion behind her, a resident slowly making her way towards the elevator. The lady's crooked body came in and out of my vision like a teeter-totter as she rocked the top half of her body back and forth to propel her wheelchair; one foot was crossed over the other on the linoleum floor.

Shifting my gaze back to this coworker, whom I knew mostly from lunch breaks, I noticed her mouth was still moving. She was still talking to me.

"I mean for the kids, it's so much more stable for your boys," she continued, as if this line of conversation made perfect sense to her.

Unable to formulate a response, my mind simply wondered away from the dim hallway and the smiling coworker and landed on images of me alone with Henry and Arthur in all kinds of different situations: traveling on a plane, struggling to set up the tent for camping. I saw Henry changing a light bulb that had just burnt out, me teaching them to ride a bike, Henry trying to fix the screen door last night after we had to cut it because I left my key in the house. Surely she did not realize how ridiculous her statement sounded. Surely it would be better if my boys could still see their dad, even just part of the time.

The ground seemed to shift beneath my feet, and I hoped there was at least a frozen smile on my face. Nothing felt stable at that moment.

"It wasn't an either/or situation." I finally replied hesitantly as the wheelchair finally turned the corner out of sight.

Shaking my head in dismay at people's lack of consideration, I proceeded down the hallway, but something about this seemingly insensitive comment kept weaving its way into my addled brain. Believing that no one is trying to be malicious in these awkward situations, I had to consider that my coworker was simply speaking her truth. No one knows what to say, so they say what they themselves think they might want to hear, or they pass along advice they think is helpful.

Contemplating her statement often as I moved forward with our lives, I realized that indeed there was comfort in knowing that all the decisions were mine. Having my children sleep in the same house every night was more stable for them. But who would spell me when I needed a break, and who could show patience with them when I had lost mine?

Parenting without a partner, making the final decision in all matters 24/7, would prove to be a blessing and a curse.

CHAPTER SIX

The Year We Invented Oatmeal

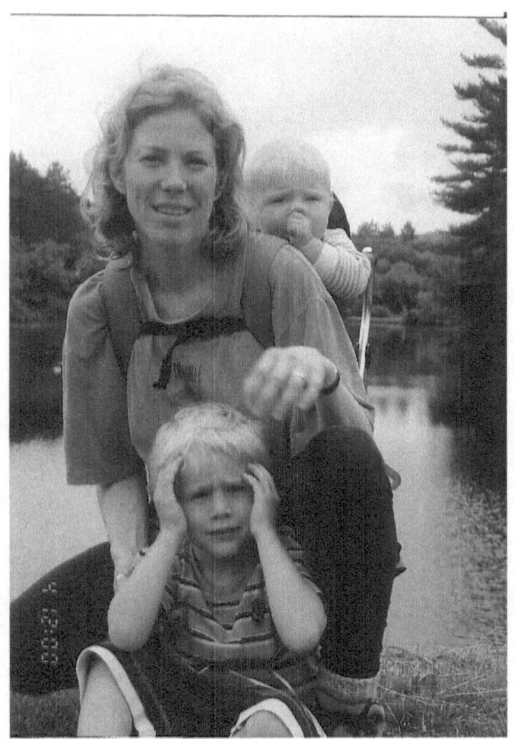

The best way out is always through.
Robert Frost

≈≈

For weeks, maybe days, maybe months, I sat Indian-style in the big chair after putting the boys to bed, surrounded by stacks of sympathy cards lined up along the thick arms of the chair. Big, oval, richly colored tulips stood proudly amongst the family pictures on top of the mantel. I read the cards one by one and vacillated between sobbing and outrage. One more card about how strong or amazing I was or that Bob was in a better place, and I was going to rip all of the sympathy cards to shreds and burn them along with all the cancer information.

Then one would tell a funny story about Bob or express the beauty they experienced at the memorial or how much they appreciated having known Bob. That's when I would cry big, heaving, gasping sobs that frightened me with their raw power, coming directly from my center and threatening to rip me in half.

There was this overwhelming feeling that a mistake had been made in the cosmos, the wrong person had died. It was not just that I didn't want to raise children by myself; I was not at all sure that I could. Bob was the one who should have been left with the boys. He was so much more natural, nurturing, and patient. How was I to obtain these qualities? We had been such a great team; I felt like Art Garfunkel of Simon & Garfunkel. Sure, I had skills and talents of my own, but I was only a big hit if Bob was by my side.

Every ounce of uncertainty and sadness and anger and regret that I had not allowed myself to acknowledge for the last year came crashing around me like an angry sea. I couldn't catch my breath before another wave hit. I felt no reason to fight these waves; control was an illusion anyway.

I knew that now.

Through the tears I had moments of clarity, like a windshield just after the wiper clears the drops of water out of its path. I could see what was important and what wasn't, if only for an instant. I felt everything so deeply. There was meaning in every tiny moment and memory. I felt so close to the truth, open and exposed, as if experiencing such profound loss put my hand on the pulse of the universe.

There was no "why", just "how" and "when".

At my first grief support group meeting (just two weeks after Bob had died), the facilitator heard all my concerns with regard to parenting. She then suggested that I might want to consider the possibility that Bob and I had made a deal with each other's energy before coming into this incarnation. We had agreed, out in the ether, that Bob would leave early and I would be left to raise the children, thus conquering my greatest fear. This deal, she continued, would explain my heightened concern about losing Bob when we were debating whether or not to have children. Somewhere in my cells, she thought, I remembered the deal that my conscious mind had let slip once I entered this lifetime.

"I would never have been that stupid," was my immediate reaction. "I would never have agreed to this plan, this is a horrible plan." I told the facilitator this with all sincerity, blue eyes glistening.

≈≈

During these purging sessions in the big chair, I grew aware of the layers of loss that I had just suffered. As if I were peeling an onion, my eyes watered with each new layer I discovered. Contrary to all my conscious thoughts of the last year, I had not only lost my co-parent. I had lost my sounding board, my cheerleader, my cook, my organizer, my philosopher, my center, my lover, my motivator, my hiking/biking/camping buddy, my best friend. The list seemed never-ending.

Opportunities for insight and meaning had been lost. The regret I felt for not having that Hallmark moment blindsided me. The remorse was devastating because I could not do anything over and do it right. A person only dies once. Did Bob have the death he wanted? I would never know. Since he never admitted to me he was dying, and I had let Bob take the lead, we had never talked about the death he wanted.

The ripples stirred by Bob's death reached far beyond my house, and I felt each one hit me like a tidal wave. A mom had lost a son, sisters and a brother had lost a sibling, nieces and nephews had lost an uncle, friends had lost a friend. Was it possible to drown while sitting in your own living room?

Bob had made me a better person. Had the best of me died with Bob? I was most certainly not the same person I was when we were together, before he got sick.

What about the boys? Did they even know what they had lost? Could I handle triple the grief, my own plus theirs? Would Henry remember his dad? How could I carry on and provide these boys with everything Bob would have given them?

I was afraid that big chair might collapse under the weight of all of this mourning and wondering, break right through the cherry wood floor and land on the hard, cold basement tiles. How long could I remain curled in the fetal position until someone came and discovered me here, shriveled and dehydrated? Many nights I woke up in the middle of the night, my neck kinked from being crunched into the arm of the big chair, my eyes blinking at the single bulb from the lamp beside me. I forced myself to hoist my body to my bedroom. It might as well have been Everest.

No, I would have never agreed to this.

≈≈

Banging ceramic bowls and measuring cups around the kitchen, I peered at Henry through dry swollen eyes as I plopped the Bisquick box down on the counter. It seemed to pulse, scornful of its very existence in my kitchen. Oh, how I resented that Bisquick box, for its mere presence in the house reminded me of all that was wrong with our severed family. I couldn't even follow Bob's famous pancake recipe.

Wanting to foster the cooking gene in Henry now that Bob was gone, I doggedly went about the morning routine Bob had established. Henry and I made pancakes together, just as he and Bob had. My motivation was fueled by resentment, though, and I could taste it in the food. Everything tasted like cardboard and had the same sharp edges going down.

I tried to explain this morning scene to my support group, sparsely filled with women in similar situations. I had found a program for children who had experienced a significant loss. It was based on the Dougie Center in Portland, a center for grieving children. While the children met with volunteers one-on-one, the adults met in a separate room. Most of the time, as I closed the door behind me and walked toward one of the brown La-Z-Boy chairs set up in a circle, I could still hear Henry screaming on the other side of the door. His separation anxiety had increased. But I endured because I was much more in need of the support than he was.

So, after I dramatized this hideous morning scene to the group, the facilitator suggested that I might not want to spend so much effort replacing Bob. She stunned me into silence by this suggestion. Then she went on—if I spent so much time and energy trying to be Bob, who was being Irene?

"You don't want your children to lose both of you, do you?" she gently prodded.

Were those bells and whistles I heard? Had a light just turned on above my head? I did not want my children to lose both of us, and it was becoming increasingly obvious that I could not be Bob. I had to discover what I brought to the table to offer these boys. I had to be genuine with my desires and actions, stop thinking in terms of what I should be.

Theory is always so much easier than reality. I couldn't turn off the negative thoughts once I returned home. They had gathered too much force to cease without a fight. Finally some little neuron connected to another, and it came to me that I should start a success journal. Journaling had helped Bob, and maybe it could help me too. I decided I would write down every positive thing I could think of that I had done that day. Maybe seeing my actions in black and white would provide me some proof that good things were indeed happening.

So, cross-legged, back in the big chair with the stacks of cards down to a few and the names on my thank-you list crossed off, I carefully smoothed out the blank page before me, wrote the date, and tapped the pen to my lips as I thought. A cup of chamomile tea steamed beside me for inspiration.

April 29, 2004

Bob has been gone one month.

Successes:

1. Kids are alive and safe in their beds.

April 30, 2004

1. Kids are alive and safe in their beds.
2. I fed them.

May 1, 2004

1. The kids are alive and safe in their beds.
2. I fed them.
3. The tea has no vodka in it.

Well, it was a start.

≈≈

Initially my family continued their rotations so that I was not alone for more than a few weeks at a time. My brother, Mike, and his wife, Kate, were the first in the rotation after the memorial. Kate is a child psychologist with a sorority girl smile and energy to match. Everyone is her best friend. The two are an interesting exercise in balance. Mike can seem reserved, even detached until he comes up against something he knows is wrong either in action or belief, and then his redheaded temper comes out to play. As his little sister, I grew up doing my best to avoid seeing that side of him.

Having lost my spouse, I knew something that no one else in my family knew. I felt suddenly ahead of all of them in a life skill. As the youngest child, I had yearned to be the first in my family to do something, anything.

Be careful what you wish for.

Actively looking for a new home at the time of their visit, I went to look at one highly recommended by the aunts. While touring the house, I learned from the owner that she had been widowed young, three years earlier. She had seen Bob's obituary in the paper and went on to tell me how she had just remarried and was selling so that she and her son and her new husband could start their new life.

Blindly I ran for the front door and cried through the whole rainy walk back to my house. "Start our new life," she had said, sounding so happy. I liked my old life; I had no interest in a new one.

≈≈

"Mommy, what is the green square thing at the bottom of the urinal?" Henry asked as we boarded the plane.

"What green thing, Babe?" I replied, distracted. I was trying to get a squirming, newly crawling Arthur settled on my lap.

The three of us were headed to visit my sister, Kathy, in Dallas. She had invited us down to hang out by their pool. Because I feared that I might never travel again, I had decided to take her up on her offer. Get back up on that horse as soon as possible, I told myself, before I had too much time to think about what I was agreeing to. With Arthur mobile now, taking the boys on a plane was not going to get any easier any time soon, so I figured I would just jump in with both feet.

I had enlisted help from my boss to get us to the airport and as far as the security checkpoint. The new security restrictions since 9/11 did not make security inspections easy on parents of young children, particularly when the ratio was one parent to two kids. The task of getting the child out of the stroller, folding the stroller up and lifting it onto the belt while holding the seven-month-old on one hip and simultaneously making sure that the three-year-old was not wandering away was enough to deter many travelers.

We had successfully made it to the gate where Henry announced that he needed to go to the bathroom and refused to go into the ladies' room with me.

"I'm a boy, Mom," he told me, as if that should explain everything.

He seemed to make it in and out fine, and I was feeling quite proud of myself as we boarded the plane. Then the question of the green square came up. What is the green square? Why is it there? What goes on in those men's bathrooms? I thought of my friend, Jim, and his comments about men's bathrooms and how disgusting they always were, compared to women's bathrooms.

My old friend, panic, was back.

Shit, I am so ill-equipped to be raising these boys on my own. I don't even know what the green square at the bottom of the urinal is. Do all urinals have these, or is there something weird about the airport bathroom? I guess I can't have him go into bathrooms on his own anymore, lest there be more questions that I can't answer ...or, worse, he could come out with the green square in question. Henry might just have to use the women's bathroom until he is at least twelve.

Henry was still looking at me expectantly as the plane took off, waiting for his answer.

"I don't know, sweetie." I tried to sound calm rather than unsure and dejected. "We can ask your Uncle Magell when we get to Dallas. He's a boy. I'm sure he'll know."

If I didn't have all the answers to these boy questions, I would surround Henry and Arthur with men who did. That was something I could do.

≈≈

Sitting on the edge of the sandbox, I watched Henry play with the tow truck while I tried to keep Arthur's pudgy little hands from sticking sand in his mouth again. We had come to the park with our play group.

Nine weeks. I counted on my sandy fingers. *It had been nine weeks.*

Thoughts of dinner kept popping into my brain. The children needed to be fed, but what? How many days in a row could a person serve instant oatmeal? (With pre-cut carrots thrown on the table for color and to fool myself that I was offering some kind of nutrition)

It's official, I can't do this. What will I have for my success journal tonight? Today is turning into a two-chai day for sure.

I was still recovering from the screaming match Henry and I had this morning over whether or not the men who "took care of Daddy" had zipped him up in a black bag before wheeling him out of the house. I honestly had no memory of that moment. Poor Henry was so desperate for me to remember it, and I was unable to simply tell him; "Yes, I remember when they zipped Daddy up in that black bag."

Henry came up with these thoughts at the oddest moments. Just when I wasn't thinking about IT for a minute, he would come out with some profound statement about how much I must miss talking with Daddy. "You guys always really liked talking with each other," he would say very matter-of-factly.

The other day we had been at the library inquiring about my book group book for the month. Arthur was in the stroller and Henry was on my hip as we watched the librarian work her magic on the computer. The familiar earthy scent of well-worn book pages calmed me.

"My daddy died," Henry said to the librarian, turning to give her the Henry Stare.

She looked at me helplessly over Henry's head, wordlessly asking, "How do you want me to respond?"

"It's true, his daddy died," I told her, nodding and shrugging my shoulders as if to say, "Don't count on me to get you out of this, lady. I've got enough of my own problems." As I kissed the top of Henry's head, a quick whiff of lavender left over from his bath reminded me to breathe deeply.

That day at the park, sitting with my chin between my knees, I shook my head and berated myself. *I'm a wreck, I'll be lucky to get to*

#4 today in my success journal. Everyone else hanging out at the park appeared to be discussing nursing and sleeping and potty training as if these topics were all there was in the world.

While ranting silently to myself, I noticed a hawk sitting on the fence about a hundred yards from the sandbox. It seemed like the most normal thing in the world that this hawk was there. My first reaction was to try and point it out to Bob before he pointed it out to me. He always pointed out hawks to me. It became a joke between us because I had never noticed hawks before meeting him. Every time he pointed one out to me, it was like the first time he saw one.

"Renie, there's a hawk," he would say, waving a finger to the sky. Bob always looked enviously at these solitary birds, as if he would like to switch places and observe life from their distant height.

Keeping my thoughts to myself, I watched the hawk serenely watch the activities at the park. At one point we made eye contact, and all of a sudden, my agitated, swirling thoughts settled as if through a funnel, and I felt rooted and solid on the Earth in a way I hadn't since Bob had died.

Positive thoughts came rushing to my mind as if uncorked. *Maybe I could do this. Look at the three of us; we are at the park on a marvelous early summer day, and we're surrounded by friends.* The boys looked healthy and somewhat happy as they dug in the sand. The sand felt warm and fine under my feet, and I could smell the muted, sweet scent of late-blooming lilacs.

"Is that a hawk?" exclaimed Catherine, pointing toward the splash pool where the hawk remained on the wire fence and taking me out of my reverie. Catherine was tall and slender and very deliberate in her movements. One long finger was pointing towards the bird, and with the other hand she shielded her eyes from the sun.

"Isn't that amazing? It's so close!" she continued, arm still outstretched.

Keeping quiet, I stared at that bird, afraid that if I took my eyes from it I would lose this grounded, confident sensation that had so solidly filled my core and once again spin into orbit.

Later, at home, I couldn't stop thinking about the hawk and the sense of calm I got when it looked at me. *If Bob could visit me from wherever he was, it would be as a hawk.* He would know that I would understand that messenger and the connection Bob had with the hawk when he was alive. Logically, I did not accept this idea at all. Thus far, I had been unable to have any kind of conversation with Bob since he died because I had no concept of him being anywhere.

I wanted very much to believe that we would see each other again in heaven. I longed for the comfort people must feel when they believe that. But I just couldn't. I knew Bob did not believe this when he was alive, and I could not make that leap either; I never could, even as a small child. Any conversation I would have with Bob now would feel silly and contrived.

I desperately wanted to talk to him, though—so desperately! Henry was right. I missed talking to him.

Thinking about the hawk as I ripped open the oatmeal packets, nearly gagging on the puff of sugar and oats from the bag, I heard the phone ring. It was Catherine, who just wanted to tell me that as she and another mom were leaving the park, they had talked about feeling Bob's presence there that day.

My heart fluttered in my chest, and I heard the secret whispering to me again. It was more friend than foe now.

"*Talk*," it said.

Instead of the over-familiar big chair, after the boys were in bed that night, I went outside and sat in a camping chair under the stars. Looking up at the sky sprinkled with stars, I wondered where Bob would go if he had the entire universe to choose from. Why would he be "watching over us" as people frequently told me he was? We must seem pretty darn boring, compared to the universe.

"Bob," I started shyly, afraid a neighbor might hear. "Stop in every once in a while, OK? I know it must be amazing out there, but I'm really floundering here and could really use your help."

The next night I got bolder.

"Bob, you can't just flit around out there and not think of us back here in the muck. I know you can't just watch us all the time, not with the whole universe out there and all, but you can't have all the fun, you have to help me. Please, help me."

The next night it all came out, I couldn't have stopped if I had wanted to, much like projectile vomiting.

"I'm sorry, Bob, I'm so sorry. I'm sorry I never asked you how it felt to know you were dying. I'm sorry I wasn't able to listen to your answer even if I'd asked. I'm sorry we didn't have more time together. I'm sorry it seemed to take all my efforts to put one foot in front of the other and take care of the boys. I'm sorry I wasn't there when you died. I'm sorry I failed you as your caregiver in Nebraska. I'm sorry I'm so practical. I'm sorry I was so immersed in my own reality."

"But you know what, Bob?" I continued, coming to this conclusion at the same time I threw it out to the universe. "There's nothing wrong with being realistic, is there? You would be the first one to tell me that. You would have assured me of that if you had been more conscious in Nebraska. Being optimistic in Nebraska would have made me too vulnerable, and I couldn't afford vulnerability at that time. I was already pregnant, a most vulnerable state. I see clearly now that being realistic was not the same as being negative, as I felt everyone implied with their pep talks. Being realistic is actually the safest thing for your emotions. That is what you knew all along, Bob, wasn't it? Being realistic gives you successes. I was too scared to be optimistic in Nebraska, Bob. At least reality was something tangible, something with a 'to do' list that I could check off."

Talking to Bob felt great. He allowed me to say out loud what the voices in my head had been whispering for months, and he gave me the answers I needed, just as he always had.

≈≈

My biggest regret in those first months after his death was that I had never asked Bob if it was OK to read his journals. There was a part of me that had never recovered from my guilt about peeking into one of them early in our relationship. Since that confession, I had respected his privacy and had tried not even to look at the cover of the closed notebook when he left it on an end table or desk.

I so wanted to read his journals now. I wanted to read about how I was the best thing that ever happened to him, how wonderful and amazing I was. But what if he confessed to feelings for another woman, or a man? What if he wrote that I wasn't really all that great—what had he been thinking when he married me? He had kept these journals since high school. Did I want to read about his previous girlfriends?

Eventually, I rationalized that he knew he was dying and that he could have destroyed the journals, so he must have left them here for a reason. Besides, after all, he was dead. So one late night I crawled into the attic and pulled out the metal file folder where Bob kept all of his spiral notebooks, all dated and in order. I pulled out one, dated September 20, 1998–June 12, 2001. Considering possible consequences, I caressed the cover of the notebook, conjuring up images of Bob in his La-Z-Boy with a red and blue fleece blanket over his legs and a caramel-colored latte in a pint glass next to him. Slowly, I opened the notebook; his familiar slanted print with the long tail on the *y* and the vertical swoosh to the *g* gave me a swift kick to the gut.

The first page I opened to was this poem.

Sept. 22, 1998

I'm looking out at mountains
where I will meet a woman
named Irene.
They are beautiful mountains
like Irene.
I am thinking of when we will
meet.
I miss her now and wish
we would be together
sooner.
I am by the ocean listening
to the waves crash constantly.
Saturday, I will meet Irene,
across the street
from the ocean.

≈≈

A high school girlfriend invited the boys and me and another friend to her parents' "cottage" in Door County, the Cape Cod of the Midwest. By "cottage", I mean a five-bedroom house with heated tile floors, a wraparound stone porch complete with Adirondack furniture and a hammock, enormous picture windows that look out at Lake Michigan, and a raised wooden path through the dunes to the lake.

Lots of crazy, drunken memories were made at this cottage, and we were there during this hot July weekend to make some more. Well, maybe not drunken this time; five children under the age of five and one pregnant lady really put a crimp in our style.

The weekend started with the discovery of a tick on my back, living there since our trip to my sister-in-law's family "farm" the week before. And when I say "farm", well …

I had successfully kept the three of us busy with out-of-town plans for much of the summer. Friends and family had been very accommodating in providing us with places to go. It helped to be surrounded by people who loved us in a place that was not our home. Bob's absence seemed less obvious somehow. I could pretend he had simply stayed at home, waiting for our return.

In Door County, my obsession with the hawk continued. Since that first sighting at the park, I had been spotting them everywhere. Each sighting seemed significant and coincidental at the same time. Looking out at the gray waters of Lake Michigan, I begged for a sign, some kind of sign that I was not crazy, that I really could take comfort in the hawk. I asked the cosmos to send me a hawk that weekend—*please, Bob, visit me here! Prove to me you are really out there, watching.*

And then it happened. The sky was turning mauve over the lake while the sun quickly sank on the opposite side of the dunes. I could smell meat browning for dinner as I slid open the screen door and stepped outside into the warm breeze. The lone bird seemed to come out of nowhere, gliding over the dunes and landing atop a telephone pole at the next cottage down. There it perched, slowly moving its head back and forth, observing the gentle waves.

"Is that a hawk? Is that a hawk?" I yelled for my girlfriends, urgently pointing at the bird, hoping for confirmation.

"I don't know. I think so. I would have to see it fly," responded one of the ladies from behind me.

That was more than enough confirmation for me. I didn't take my eyes off that bird until it flew away, gliding out over the lake and into the ether.

≈≈

Breaking the rule against big changes for a year after the death of a spouse, I bought a new home. Buying the new house was the easy part; selling the old one was another story. We moved to our three-bedroom bungalow directly across from the grade school just four months after Bob died, following a flurry of activity by my dad: organizing and reorganizing Bob's tools, having garage sales, and making trips to the secondhand book store. The new place was painted and cleaned, thanks to family and friends. We settled quite nicely into the new neighborhood, which was full of young children and helpful neighbors.

Unfortunately the old house wouldn't sell, and I hated the idea of it being empty and alone. One day I had to swing by the old house before picking the boys up from day care to make sure everything was OK for a viewing. I meant to make sure the lawn didn't need mowing and perhaps boil some lavender oil on the stove. I parked on the street so I could go up the front walk, wanting to see the house the way the perspective buyer would see it. From the sidewalk, I could see something on the steps leading up to the porch. It looked like a sidewalk chalk drawing.

As I got closer, I saw that it was a sidewalk chalking, but it was not a child's drawing. "Someone died here", it read in neat writing, with an arrow pointing toward the house in case more specific information was needed.

I had to get on my knees with a bucket to scrub the offensive words off the sidewalk. *Who would do this to me? Where would one rather die? Assholes….!* The image of Bob in the bed in front of the fireplace with our friends and his family surrounding him as I massaged oil on his slim feet suddenly felt tainted.

I was trying to be logical about an illogical occurrence. This note was not the work of someone out to get me personally. This was the work of some young, thoughtless child. However, as I knelt there, with the concrete digging into my knees and my eyes watering from the bright sun directly overhead, the gesture sure felt personal.

Another day, leaving the boys in the car, I ran in the old house and went right to the basement to get the vacuum that we had left there. Hearing a thump upstairs, I thought Henry must have come in from the car. Dragging the vacuum up the stairs, I left it by the back door and went to look for Henry.

Walking through the kitchen, I peered into the empty dining room, which looked so big with no table and chairs, and saw no sign of him. I continued up the three steps to the landing at the bottom of the stairs and proceeded back down the other three to the foyer. Heading toward the living room, something askew caught my eye. There were some long pieces of wood leaning against the wall next to the front door.

Hmm, that's weird. Did I have someone doing some work here?

Then I noticed the front door, slightly ajar, and my heart began to thump. Looking back at the pieces of wood, I realized that there was an entire pane of glass missing to the right of the front door.

"Damn it!" My cry echoed in the cavernous house. "The stained glass, the bastards have stolen my stained glass!" My worst fear about leaving the house unoccupied had come true. Not thinking the thieves might still be in the house I dashed out the front door and yelled to my neighbor across the street. As luck would have it, he happened to be outside.

He came running, almost as distraught as I was. Soon the police were there, along with the aunts and Sarah and Garrett, whom I had called for diapers as well as support. The boys were now inside, Arthur was crawling around the bare floor, and Henry was silent and wide-eyed as the adults around him loudly cursed.

The good news was that the vandals had only gotten away with one pane of glass. The bad news was that I think I walked in on them in the middle of their "work". That might have been the thumping noise from the basement that I had thought was Henry. At least three other windows, including the gorgeous grapevine design above the built-in china cabinet, showed signs of vandals' work.

"I will never sell this house now," I wailed. "Who's going to want this house now?" I kept repeating, leaning over the counter, head in my hands, as the others tried to comfort me amidst their own dismay. "I need to have a house clearing. That is what I need. Someone needs to come in here and burn some sage or something."

And that was what just what I did.

≈≈

Watching the man approach the back door, I couldn't help but be a little skeptical. Jeff had a long, graying beard and hair and a worn leather jacket and jeans. He might have just come from a Harley rally or a ZZ Top concert. But he had kind eyes and a gentle energy about him and had come highly recommended by a friend of mine, someone with whom I exchanged massages.

Jeff told me he wouldn't burn sage due to the open house scheduled for the next day, but he walked around the house, mumbling to himself and placing crystals strategically throughout.

I followed him nervously from room to room and babbled that I thought maybe Bob did not want me to sell the house. Maybe he was lurking about, scaring people away. But Jeff assured me it was not Bob and that Bob was not here. There was not a lot of bad energy in this house, he said, reassuring me. Just a "little something" in the computer room, Jeff said, probably left over from when this house was a burial ground for the Native Americans who once lived here, and it was nothing bad.

As we walked into the basement and the room that Bob had used as his bike shop, I thought how sad it looked without the bike stand and the familiar upside-down bike that usually adorned the room. No tools lined up along the counter. The brown speckled linoleum had never looked this bad with bicycle tires and tools strewn over it.

"Oh, this is it," the medium said in an *ah ha* tone. His shoulders relaxed a bit, and he looked wistfully around the room.

"This is where Bob liked to spend his time. He felt most himself here," Jeff continued, more to himself than me.

"He worked on his bikes here," I said awkwardly before launching into a string of questions. "Is he OK? Is he happy? Does he visit me as a hawk? Were we soul mates? Will there be anyone else for me?"

The medium responded patiently to my tirade. Yes, Bob was OK. Yes, he could visit me as a hawk, and I might even feel him physically in the room at times. I would most likely begin to take on some of his characteristics. (His cooking skills, I thought, would be good.) Jeff explained that "soul mate" was a misused term. Twin flames are what most people think of as soul mates. A soul mate is anyone you have agreed to have a connection with over the course of your life. It could be as simple as someone you meet at the airport who helps you get to the correct plane, or it could be your best friend through college.

"Were Bob and I twin flames?" I asked, already knowing the answer. "Will I see him again as someone or something else?"

"Yes, you two had lived lives together before," Jeff told me. "But he won't come back again while you're still here in this same incarnation. He'll wait where he is."

"Bob didn't believe any of what you are talking about when he was alive," I told him.

"He does now," Jeff retorted, as surely as if Bob were in the room telling him so.

I continued my questioning…But what if … but what if …

With one hand on the door, trying to leave, the medium looked me right in the eye. "Renie, don't worry," he said, and the tone was perfect!

I stared, waiting for Bob to emerge from beneath the mask this man must be wearing. The air around me seemed lighter, and my breathing felt easy. Taking a deep breath for the first time in what seemed like months, I felt my ribcage expand and welcome the oxygen. I felt calm and assured in the knowledge that Bob was within me, not gone. I carried him always. I could move forward without his physical presence because I brought all that he was with me now.

The message seemed clear—don't worry. It will all be revealed in time.

The house clearing was the single most beneficial thing I had done for myself since Bob died. Faith is all about semantics, and I had finally heard the right words.

Jeff took one last look at the house before walking to his car.

"Someone wants this house," he told me. "They are close by."

The house sold the next day to a young widow who had been staying with her brother-in-law down the block.

≈≈

I stopped at the old house on the way to the closing, went straight upstairs to the top floor, and sat down with my back up against the closet door. Looking out the window, I remembered sitting in the rocking chair while nursing Henry. Slowly rocking back and forth, I would look alternately at Henry's perfect ears and the perfect leaves on the oak tree as they turned a dusty red. Sometimes we would see Bob drive up the street, back from work, and I would feel my relief at his arrival in my stomach.

The house, by then, was always ready for a little "Bob energy". Soon the smell of dinner would fill the house, and the steady routine of the evening would begin. Perhaps we would enjoy a bike ride, a walk in the neighborhood, or a trip to the lakefront, where huge telescopes were available for stargazing. Bob always knew when Saturn's rings were visible or Mars was the closest it would be to the Earth for the next two hundred years.

There was no point in looking out that window now. Bob was never coming home, and I could really use some Bob energy right now. I lay down on the stiff brown carpeting and stared at the slanted ceiling and the window on the north side. Once a bat got stuck in the plant that covered that window like a curtain. Bob had told me calmly to walk down to the guest room. "Why?" I insisted. When the situation became obvious to me, that the rustling and squeaking coming from the plant was indeed not the rain, I threw the covers over my head and yelled for Bob to do something about it.

Then I pictured Bob standing at his dresser getting ready for work. Snuggled in our bed, I often watched him pick out his clothing from the long dark dresser he had from his youth. Often he danced a goofy dance while he chose the clothes, a cross between Elaine from *Seinfeld* and John Travolta in *Saturday Night Live*. Rolling my eyes and chuckling a bit, I would pull the covers up around my chin, roll over, and go back to sleep.

I wasn't supposed to be sitting here in an empty house that I was about to sign over to another family. We were supposed to be raising our children here. The boys were supposed to come find you in the morning, Bob, and finger all the mysterious treasures on the top of your dresser while you performed your silly dance for them. They were supposed to spot your car from that window and yell, "Dad's home!" We were all supposed to laugh at the bat memory, so ensconced in our family lore by repeated telling at the dinner table that the boys would believe they had actually been there to see Mom cower under the covers while Dad took a tennis racket to the swooping animal.

I rolled on my side and curled up, knees to chest, turning my back on the memories. The carpet felt scratchy against my cheek as the tears silently slid across my nose and dripped onto the carpet so fast they pooled there before they could be absorbed. *What if* and *should have been* bombarded me as I huddled in the fetal position and ultimately surrendered to big, heaving sobs.

"I'm sorry, Bob!" I told him as my crying echoed in the empty room. "I'm so sorry. I just can't keep this house." Pounding the carpet, I continued, "I can't give our boys the life we planned in this house. I just can't without you. I wish I could. I'm so sorry, Bob. I'm so sorry," I repeated until the sobs subsided. Then I lay on my back again, drawing in unsteady breaths.

"It's OK. We're OK, right?" I finally concluded. "The new house is good. It's actually the three-bedroom bungalow I always wanted, Bob, ironic, huh? You didn't have to die for me to get the house I wanted. That was a little extreme."

I began to laugh uncontrollably. The absurdity of crawling around the floor while apologizing to Bob and joking about how far he would go to give me what I wanted struck me as insanely humorous, or just insane.

Emboldened and restored, I stood up and walked out without looking back. I walked through each room briefly. Then I headed out the back door, closed it behind me, got in the car, drove to the meeting, and signed the papers with tears bright in my eyes and a hesitant grin on my face.

≈≈

In the checkout line at the natural food co-op, my body felt tense and springy. I had just been across the street at the grocery store and stood in line behind an older couple who bickered about which carton of cigarettes to buy. They were a depressing sight. Both of them were overweight and sallow; their hair lank and greasy. In their cart was every processed food imaginable, a box of Twinkies on top like a cherry on a sundae.

My resentment boiled beneath my skin. "They will probably live to be a hundred," I muttered under my breath. The man was probably an absentee dad—I was sure of it. I was caustic and cynical about everything these days, it seemed. For any story about a deadbeat dad, any wife overheard complaining about her husband, or any TV commercial about someone being cured of cancer by prayer, I had a sarcastic comeback all ready.

As I waited in line, I hoped that the co-op had fixed the ownership paperwork and that I wouldn't have to see "Bob Wellenstein" on my receipt as I had every time I shopped in this store since his death. I had tried to fix this issue several different times, and each time the person told me it was taken care of. Then, the next time I shopped, I would find that it was not. I'd see "Bob Wellenstein" on my receipt. I had been told that I had to bring in proof of his death—seriously, proof of his death—for the community co-op. We are talking about $2.00 in dividends each year.

I had even offered to bring in the urn.

The poor, unsuspecting checkout guy looked like he was sixteen. With a short military haircut and a fresh face, he probably didn't need to shave. He pleasantly bagged groceries for the customer in front of me, blissfully ignorant of the storm that was brewing with his next customer.

He grabbed my first item off the belt, smiling, and asked for my member number. "*16559*," I answered. I felt a bit nauseated with anxiety about what would come next. Here it came …

"Bob Wellenstein?" he asked cheerfully after inputting the number.

"NO!" I erupted. He stared at me, shocked and mute. "Look, I've been trying to get his name off the account for months now. I know it's not YOUR fault." I attempted politeness. "But why can't you people get his name off my account?"

"You will have to go to customer service," the boy politely told me.

"I have been to customer service! I have filled out forms. I have written letters. I have had friends call for me, they have written letters. What more do you people want from me? My husband died! I offered to bring in the urn as proof! But you people can't seem to get him off my account. I don't want to have to see his name on every goddamn receipt every goddamn time I come in here to buy some food."

From the corners of my bulging eyes, I could see the customer behind me quickly removing his items from the belt and putting them gingerly back in his cart, tiptoeing to another checkout line.

My body shook, my face was red, there was spittle coming out of my mouth, and I think I even saw the checkout boy brush the spray from his face. I didn't care. I felt completely justified. My request was not outrageous or difficult. I simply wanted a name off my membership, which should take no more than a push of a computer button.

"Ma'am, this is equity," they had told me. There were "procedures". I just wanted to shop at my local grocery store without having my dead husband's name thrown at me each time. They were the ones being unjust, not me. Of that I was certain.

My anger phase was purged all over that baby-faced checkout boy. I could only imagine the next staff meeting.

I never saw him at that store again.

I never saw Bob's name on another receipt either.

≈≈

"You have to stop coughing," I pleaded with Henry. It was one in the morning, and the two of us stood in the middle of the too-bright kitchen. My hands gripped his shoulders, and I looked straight into his bleary blue eyes.

Arthur's first birthday was the next day, and I was having the family over for cake. I was recovering from a cold, that ugly stage where you are clearing your lungs and coughing up unpleasant slimy things. It was my first illness since Bob had been diagnosed, and it had filled me with terror, the irrational kind. It was just a cold, but I felt so much pressure to stay well for the boys that my mind went to ugly, dark places.

To make things worse Henry had his usual seasonal cough, deep and seal-like. The two of us had been gargling with tea tree oil, taking lavender baths, and drinking lemon and honey tea until I was afraid we might just float away on a yummy smelling current. This was day four of being up in the middle of the night, and I was exhausted and apparently out of my mind.

"Really, please, you have to stop coughing," I continued, shaking his shoulders lightly. Some part of me knew this demand was not rational. How could I be standing here in this kitchen while begging my four-year-old to stop coughing, as though his cough were poor behavior on his part? How dare he have a cough? Didn't he know I wasn't feeling well? Didn't he know I was overwhelmed and unhappy? Couldn't he just stop coughing … for me … please?

A few days later, I confessed to a coworker about that night. "That's just not right," I told her. "I think I might be losing it."

"You're tired, Irene," she said. "Don't be so hard on yourself."

Was I being too hard on myself? Or was I actually falling apart? It seemed a fine line at this point.

≈≈

"God damn it, Bob," I cried aloud toward the heavens. "I miss the smell of dinner cooking when I get home from work. God damn you. Spoiling me like that, with all your creative recipes and pure joy in the kitchen. Fuck you, leaving me here to feed the three of us on my own. It's not like I don't know how to cook, you know, but I just can't live up to the way you cooked for us. And oh, how I miss the way you cooked for us!" I began to pace around the kitchen and mumble under my breath. "I can't get a decent meal on the table, Bob. Shit, it's all I can do to have two clean sippy cups for the boys to have their smoothies in the morning. And if I haven't made up the smoothie before I go to bed, then I am screwed for the morning." Collapsing onto a stool, I put my head in my hands and continued to whimper softly. "I am pathetic. Bob, really, shit, I need some help here … please."

Unraveling, unhinging, falling apart. That was what I was doing, right before the boys' eyes in the middle of the kitchen amidst the diaper bag, my briefcase, Henry's canvas school bag, and a brown grocery bag full of frozen food. All of these items quietly remained where I dropped them upon our entry to the house.

Henry quietly assessed the situation, sighed heavily, and marched into the dining room. There he proceeded to take a role of Scotch tape and mummify a flannel blanket to our dining room chair, a new activity I found fascinating and disturbing at the same time. Arthur, having just learned to walk, teetered off behind him, unfazed by the scene of his mother being hysterical in the kitchen. He had seen it all before.

Arthur proceeded to remove the tape that Henry was working so diligently on and then the screaming ensued, and the chasing, and the grabbing.

I remained fixed in the kitchen, just hoping the two of them would wear themselves out before someone got hurt.

Bob had been gone eight months now, and this was an all too familiar scene for me these days. I was just home from work and seemingly unable to put together a meal for the three of us that didn't consist of something frozen or ordered. I had hardly progressed at all from the days of instant oatmeal. I felt sick. No, I felt hollow, as if someone had taken a cold ice cream scoop to my rib cage. I felt too skinny; a strong breeze might be all it would take to knock me down.

I didn't just miss the smell of the house when Bob was alive and did the cooking. I missed the feel of the house too. The frequent simmering of garlic and ginger, the sizzling of pancakes, the gentle clink of the whisk against the bowl, all the cooking smells and sounds coming from the kitchen filled the house with a dense, warm air that made those drafty old rooms feel cozy. Now the house felt cold and sterile, like a hospital cafeteria, and anything I cooked tasted about as good as hospital food.

Sarah even bought me a crock pot with the idea that I could come home and the house would be filled with the delicious smell of a slow-cooked meal. But the first evening the three of us sat down to eat the pot roast I had so painstakingly prepared, Henry cried and refused to eat it because the meat was touching the potatoes. Arthur simply sat in his high chair and threw tiny meat pieces on the floor. The meal ended with Henry fixing his own peanut butter and jelly sandwich and me crying while I envisioned the next ten years of my life involving dinners just like this one.

Wretched, that was how I felt. The people who told me I was strong and too hard on myself never saw these scenes. I was convinced all over again that the wrong person had died. The boys should have been left with Bob if they had to be left with just one of us; at least then they would still be eating well.

"OK, OK, Irene, you have to get yourself together," I said out loud, shaking my head and patting my cheeks to clear the haze that was closing in. "You can do this. You love to bake, and you make fabulous spaghetti sauce. A person can live on banana bread and noodles, right?"

Clawing at my throat, I was barely breathing. I was thinking of never having ginger chicken again, or fried tofu, or Bob's famous pizza, or those waffles he made that one time. One more dinner of frozen chicken nuggets and macaroni and cheese might just have me running from the house. *What were we going to do? What was I going to do?*

I heard that old familiar whisper, and it said *"cook, eat"* as if the words blew into the kitchen from the back door. Slowly I unfolded myself from the fetal position. The words surrounded me and lifted me up. Before I knew what was happening, I found my hand reaching into the cabinet toward Bob's recipe file.

I needed a goal. I made a decision. I felt inspired.

Quickly I warmed water on the stove and made instant oatmeal for the boys. Just one more night I told myself. I got them to bed, cleaned the kitchen, packed a snack for Henry for school the next day, took out the garbage, got bottles ready for Arthur, and made the smoothie for the morning. Then I sat on the stool in front of the stove and slowly went through Bob's files and picked out my favorite five recipes that he had made for us.

Silently I wept when I found the cranberry chicken recipe he had made for my last birthday with him. The deep red cranberries and the bright green broccoli made the evening look a bit like Christmas. I laughed out loud when I found the African chicken recipe he had made for Sarah and Garrett one night. The dish was so hot that we all lunged for the water glasses, our eyes watering, after just one bite.

I imagined him fingering all these delicate pieces of paper that he had so carefully cut out of newspapers or magazines and filed by category. I remembered him sitting at the dining room table, scissors in hand, slowly turning the pages of the morning paper. Occasionally he would chuckle and shake his head.

"Oh, Renie, you're going to hate this one." Then he would be off to the store for saffron.

That night, alone in the kitchen, I made a pact with myself. I vowed I would make my five favorite recipes before the one-year anniversary of his death. It was now November. This goal gave me over four months to make five dishes and fill the house with the old familiar scents.

I would plan the meals for when I had family visiting and for special occasions; that way I would have motivation and assistance. I would wrap the three of us up in the soothing heat of a well-cooked meal.

I WAS strong. I could do this.

≈≈

"Irene, do you think you might want to talk to your doctor about medication?"

That was my boss, standing in front of me in my office, concern laced with pity stitched across her forehead. I was crying again. About what, I had no idea; sadness quickly switched to anger. This show of sympathy burned in my belly. *Screw you. I'm sorry my grief is so difficult to watch, but imagine living it every day. And I'm really trying to LIVE it. I HAVE to live it. I don't want to live this life. I would like to be doing anything but live with this grief, but I have no choice. I was given no choice.*

"My husband died eight months ago." I said aloud. "I don't think a pill will help me with that, unless there's a pill to bring him back. I don't want medication. I'm situationally depressed. Wouldn't it be more concerning if I wasn't depressed?" I really believed what I was saying. I was getting out of bed in the mornings. I was taking care of the boys. I was functioning.

My mourning wasn't pretty, I admit, but I had to suffer fully, really feel the sorrow, live with all the miserable and hopeless thoughts, the overwhelming sense of gloom that invaded my every move. Really feeling all of these daunting emotions with my eyes wide open was the only way to purge myself of them. If I ever hoped to live beyond the grief, I had to first live with it.

≈≈

My mother's helper started very soon after my meltdown in the kitchen. Hearing my complaints of dinner and bedtime one too many times, my sister Kathy suggested that I hire someone for the "witching hour". That meant the time from five PM until seven, those hours when the kids are tired and I am tired and food needs to get on the table and dishes need to be washed and children need baths and stories.

I had found myself hurtling through the bedtime routine so I could get my chores done and have some time to myself. There was entirely too much yelling. I had to admit I wasn't doing well on my own. I couldn't do it all—not happily. I did not make a good martyr.

Enter Paola, my savior, the best thing that happened to me in a year. When that skinny brown body and long straight wet hair entered the house that late fall day, I could sense the winds changing in my favor.

The first night she came, I sat in the big chair and read to Henry. Arthur was already asleep in his crib. I heard the familiar banging and clanking of a kitchen being cleaned. Tears of joy and relief sprang to my eyes. The heavy burden of responsibility lifted, just a little, maybe just enough.

≈≈

Arthur sat in the stroller and Henry stood beside me as we snaked our way through the security line at the Denver airport. There was the stale electric energy of people hurrying up and waiting that airports have. Christmas was finally over, and people were going back to their lives laden with packages and over-sugared children.

The line inched forward. Arthur pushed the belly of his new bear, and "We love you, Arthur," sing-songed into the crowd for the hundredth time. Henry, clutching his new tool belt Santa brought, was wide-eyed, watching the people. It seemed to me that I saw only families—couples busy keeping children occupied. I felt weak and pale and anxious, my eyes were scratchy, and I was just trying to make it to the plane without an incident.

Christmas had come, as I knew it would, and I had prepared myself for the hurdles I had to jump this first year. That meant getting our holiday photo taken with just the three of us, writing the Christmas letter, decorating the tree without my light guy, hanging up the three stockings and leaving a big gaping hole where the fourth belonged, and traveling with the two boys by myself to be with my family so I didn't have to wake up alone on Christmas morning.

I had endured the regular McGoldrick traditions of Swedish tea rings and hanging stockings and gift exchanging around the tree laden with handmade ornaments, as I would endure a trip to the dentist. I knew all that was what I needed to be doing, good for me, good for us, and necessary, but it was uncomfortable at best and painful most of the time. Aching inside, I smiled outwardly during each visit with friends as I watched the dad scoot the kids off to bed with a kiss on the forehead.

I had frequently felt as if a truck had come out of nowhere and broadsided me. Christmas cards had always been my favorite part of the holidays. This year, however, they elicited trepidation instead of enthusiasm. Forgetting that Bob had died in many people's lives and not just mine, I was shocked the first time I read about the loss in someone else's letter, as if the writer had plagiarized a part of my life. And sometimes I didn't appreciate the way the story was related. Reading a casual comment about a first plane ride for a son on the way to Bob's memorial or someone proselytizing about why it had all happened felt like a kick in the gut.

After returning from the tree-cutting ritual for which I had commandeered the aunts, I opened that first box of ornaments to find BOB staring me in the face. Hand-stitched in red yarn on his stocking by my mom a few years back, his name sat atop the rosy Santa face and the fuzzy beard. Bob had packed the boxes up the year before, probably wondering, as he folded up that stocking and carefully placed it on top of the other three, if he would be here this year to hang it above the fireplace. Staring at his name on the stocking, I could not fathom how we would manage to decorate the tree with ornaments from vacations Bob and I had taken together.

But I had successfully made it through it all and found myself at the airport, awkwardly folding up the stroller so it would fit on the security belt. Meanwhile I hoped Arthur, in his Dalmatian-spotted fleece outfit, would not take off down the concourse as he had when we left Milwaukee. I noticed an older couple, grandparent types, probably on their way home after spoiling the grandchildren for a week. They glanced at me dubiously, wondering if the scene was precious or obnoxious, as I struggled to get my shoes off, keep

Arthur from sprinting through the metal detector, and explain to Henry why he couldn't even joke about bombs in an airport. Once we arrived at our gate, I noticed the couple again, observing us as Arthur and Henry rode up and down the escalator. I was sure that they hoped these rambunctious children and their frazzled single mother wouldn't be on their plane.

The same couple sat in front of us on the plane. Arthur was mercifully sleeping and Henry was already asking how much longer the flight would be as we sat waiting to taxi to the runway. Then the pilot's voice rang out over the intercom, just a little too cheery, asking us if we were all comfortable—a very bad sign. He explained that there was some problem.(Engine? Tire? Who cared?) Whatever the reason, it meant we weren't taking off for at least two hours, and we weren't being let off the plane either. Sheer panic led me to search for the baggie of Fruit Loops my friend had thrown in my bag at the last minute, just in case, and quickly play the widow card.

"I was recently widowed," I blurted to the couple in front of me, hoping my instincts were right about the grandparent thing. "This is our first Christmas without my husband … their dad. We came to Colorado to be with my family so I wouldn't have to be alone." I stressed "alone".

I needed sympathy to get through this delay in one piece and not injure either of the boys in the process. It doesn't take long to realize that in our society, a widowed mother will get much more sympathy than a single one.

"Oh, dear, I'm so sorry," they responded in unison, expressions changing from annoyance to compassion. "Your boys are so good. You're doing such a nice job." Then a shoulder nudge to the husband—"Help her get that cereal out of her bag, honey."

I was not above playing the widow card.

Once we were finally in the air, I had time for contemplation. I couldn't stop thinking about a conversation I had with my brother, Mike, and his wife, Kate. I had spent an evening with them at their bungalow in Denver. The boys had stayed with Grandma and Grandpa, and I had relished the opportunity to sit in their living room and talk without interruptions.

The subject of marrying again came up.

"I liked being married to Bob," I said. I had read somewhere that people who had been happily married were more likely to marry again. "I don't see myself on my own for the rest of my life." This was as much wishful thinking as anything. "I mean, Bob taught me the benefit of being in a relationship, so it would be cruel to learn that and then just be left here alone, don't you think?" More wishful thinking.

"But who would want to date me?" I asked the sympathetic eyes across the coffee table. The heads began to tilt to one side, and they shifted in their chairs; sympathy could turn to pity so easily.

"I don't mean who would want to date ME, I mean who would want to take on all THIS." I gestured to signify the children, who were not there. "My children are so young. I wouldn't want to date someone in my situation."

"It wouldn't be the boys that would scare me off, Renie." Mike spoke quietly and sincerely. "It would be living up to the sainted dead husband."

Now that was a lot to think about. I filed that comment away. Bob and I did have an extremely easy relationship, we were very well suited, but he was no saint. I guess it is human nature to remember only the good things about a person once he is gone. I made a mental note to remember the good, the frustrating, and the annoying about Bob and share all these aspects with Henry and Arthur. I didn't want them to have to live up to a saint either.

≈≈

Sarah, Garrett and I were spending a spontaneous weekend sans kids in Door County at the same friend's house on Lake Michigan. Sarah spent most of the weekend knitting in front of the fire. I curled up on a couch to read, but the soft, rhythmic clicking of the needles made me feel very meditative, so I mostly stared out the huge picture window, past the snow-covered dunes where the steel-gray waves crashed steadily ashore. I was taking stock of my life—where I was, how far I had come since this time last year.

It was mid-January, the weather had been frigid, and I was careening toward the first anniversary of Bob's death. I was still attending my support group. However, I was quickly becoming more facilitator than participant, feeling ready to move past the group but also somewhat responsible to the other ladies there. My success journal regularly saw double-digit numbers now.

Henry and Arthur and I were settled into the new house, and Henry had started at a Montessori preschool that was perfect for him. The neighbors were very attentive to the widow on the block, shoveling and fixing fallen window boxes. My parents had just offered to move back to Milwaukee from Colorado to help us. (I quickly jumped on that offer!) That enormous gesture taught me more about unconditional love and the never-ending job of parenting than I cared to know at the time.

The aunts took the boys overnight so I had some time for myself and to keep up with my friends. I got regular massages and started drinking red wine. I was meticulously cooking my way through those five favorite recipes of Bob's, trying to fill the house up with the familiar smells of garlic and ginger. These rich scents seemed to fill the house with something like comfort and made my ribcage feel a bit less hollow. My goal was to not need Bisquick or instant oatmeal ever again.

Most recently I had been working with a friend who did esoteric healing, or energy work, as I called it. The good thing about not believing in something was that I felt open to anything.

Energy work was a lot like talk therapy. She came every few weeks after the kids were in bed, and we sat, facing each other, on the futon. We started each session by checking in on how my life had been going since our last meeting and talking about my intention for this session. I interpreted "intention" to mean "goal".

She often asked me to ask my "higher self" for guidance and listen for an answer. Dutifully I asked the question and sat there for an appropriate amount of time while waiting for an answer, although I never heard anything. Then I would sit in a straight-backed chair, and she would put her hands on either side of me. Never touching me, she moved her hands up a bit and down, then above my head.

Often times she would pick up on things I had been worrying about but had not mentioned during our talk, asking me if I was worried about money or health, for instance. (The weird part was that I had always been obsessing about just what she mentioned.)

And then she was done. I never felt anything physically, but she always said that I might have labile emotions for the next couple of days.

Mostly I argued with her. She would tell me I shouldn't say I was a wreck because events are the way you interpret them. She would say I shouldn't be sad and that the events of my life were happening the way they should. Like my first support group leader, this one believed that Bob and I had agreed to this situation in some other dimension. This was all that Bob could do in this lifetime. Maybe, she suggested, I had left Bob early in a previous life.

"So this is payback? Bob didn't seem the vindictive type," I would answer sarcastically.

Besides, even if I did agree to that plan, I still missed him, and what was I supposed to do about that? Aren't I trapped in my own humanity, reacting to a very real human situation with very real human emotion? Don't you have to really feel the sadness in order to be cleansed of it? Even if you sit around and envision how you want things to be and intend for them to happen, you still have to get from A to B, right?

And that is the hard part—getting there.

The hardest part of mourning is that no one else can do it for you. Friends and family can worry and care and be supportive and even help with meals or paperwork, but they can't live through each day for you. You have to get out of bed in the morning and get the boys' smoothie and go through your day without the person who made it all worthwhile. I had to discover a different purpose and worth, and I knew I would. I didn't know the exact steps I would have to take to get there.

I thought I deserved a little sadness, a little time to be a wreck and wallow. People are afraid to wallow. They are scared that they might always feel that far down in the depths and never feel lighthearted again. My bigger fear concerned *not* feeling so deeply anymore—the day I could not play the widow card, the day someone told me to move on.

I was terrified of the first day that would go by with no thought of Bob. I also feared the day when I would talk about him casually, like a college roommate I once knew, with no sharp pain in my stomach or tears in my eyes.

"Without suffering there can be no joy," the Buddhists say. I guess the point is that I should be rejoicing that I had something to grieve. "If you had nothing to grieve, that would be true sadness," I concluded to Jeanne one day on the phone while tears streamed down my face. I guess these were the labile emotions I had been warned about.

Prior to the Door County trip, I had set my latest goal with my energy worker. My goal was to enjoy the boys and not see them as only a responsibility. I knew we had to become a more cohesive family. A few days earlier, while waiting in line to drop Henry off at school, a mom and dad got out of the car in front of us to bring their daughter up to the door together. Henry watched them walk up to the door, all three of them, hand in hand, the parents swinging the girl between them.

"The whole family came today," Henry said wistfully, "We aren't a family anymore."

That simple statement knifed my heart.

At the next esoteric healing session, I spoke about this incident and about how I needed to do something family-oriented, something community-oriented, something with people who didn't know Bob, somewhere that I didn't have a big "W" on my forehead. When I asked my higher self that night, the word *"church"* popped into my mind.

Disillusioned young for no apparent reason, I had not been a believer since I was a young child. Mutual lack of belief in God had been a bond between Bob and me. Bob was the scientist, always needing proof. We were able to find our own version of spirituality in nature and travel.

"Church" had become a word with a negative connotation for me. I had to sit with the idea for a while. What would my friends say?

While in Door County that wintry weekend, Sarah and I went to a spa for massages. We sat in a steam room beforehand. My skin, dry from the cold and the forced air in the house, soaked up the moist heat, and I began to feel plumped up.

"I'm thinking of going to church," I said slowly, as if making a confession. I thought I should try out the word to take some of the sting out of it. Next I would try "worship". "I was thinking about the Unitarian church."

That was always the only one Bob said he could handle, and I thought that any church with services titled, "What the Simpsons Have to Teach Unitarian Universalists" and "Everything Jesus Said about Homosexuality" might be the place for me.

"I just need a place where we can go as a family," I tried to explain, more for me than for her.

"I think that's a good idea," Sarah responded supportively, trying to keep any shock out of her voice.

So off we went to church the next weekend, when my sister Anne was in town. She had come for my birthday. Nothing ruffled that woman's feathers, even after I told her my plan to bring Bob (in the urn, of course) to our usual birthday dinner restaurant with the usual couples. The idea of church seemed rather normal after that, I am sure.

The service we attended was called "Trusting the Spirit of Life". The minister, Drew Kennedy, a fabulous orator with a practiced, measured cadence and a hairstyle that looked like it wouldn't move even in hurricane wind, spoke about basic trust, developed in the early years of life and tested again and again when people, nature, God, or technology disappointed us.

Was this minister, who had never met me, speaking directly to me when he posed this question asked by Roy Phillips, another Unitarian Universalist minister?

"Do you heavily guard and defend yourself against each misfortune and therefore miss not only what harms, but also much that brings delight?"

I had asked myself numerous times what the point of loving someone again would be. The guy would just die on me eventually, and I couldn't go through that again. Was I holding back from my kids for this same reason? Sitting arrow-straight in the wood pew, memories of childhood and frankincense surrounding me, I pondered these questions as the minister continued.

Perhaps, the minister suggested, we need to learn to trust in the darkness. Theodore Roethke said, "The dark has its own light." Personal growth and positive transformations often emerge from times of personal pain … when the darkness, with its own lessons and wisdom (light), has descended upon us. "So," Drew boomed from the pulpit, "trust in life—even its darkness."

My body felt as if it were vibrating at a low level, the hairs on my arm stood straight up. The Order of Service I was holding grew soggy from my sweaty palms.

Drew ended with a quote from a story about a dad, Philip Booth, teaching his daughter to swim,

> Remember, when fear cramps your heart …
> Lie back,
> And the sea
> will hold you.

The pianist started playing, and I sat transfixed, feeling that the sermon might have been written and delivered specifically for me. The rustle of people leaving their pews startled me. I had felt alone in the sanctuary. His words made so much sense to me.

I needed to trust in the darkness.

Lie back, and let the sea hold me.

≈≈

Kathy was assigned to the one-year anniversary of Bob's death. I had been planning this date for a year now. The boys were dropped off at day care, and the two of us went to my favorite coffee shop for a second cup of chai. Every March 29th, I declared, would be a two-chai day. In fact, any day that I needed just a little bit of extra support, a little extra love and comfort, I declared a two-chai day. Why deny myself, what was the point of such limits?

After the coffee shop, we went to get a tattoo of a hawk on my left ankle. Kathy wrinkled her nose, looking out of place in the dark room with pictures of angels and eagles hanging on the walls. Sitting neatly on a stool in her Capri's and matching blouse, she commented about all the blood on the washcloth that the artist kept swiping over the area he was intently working on. I had to remind her that I was having tiny needles repeatedly stuck in my flesh. A last-minute addition of "3/29" went below the realistic red-winged hawk, and my memorial tattoo was finished.

Kathy and I returned home for the most anticipated of the planned rituals', the reading of the letter from Bob that I had discovered the same evening he died. An entire year had been spent in anticipation of this final note to me. *What were the last words he wanted to say to me? Would they be about his enduring love? His thoughts on dying? His hopes and wishes for the boys?*

Kathy poured wine for me, and we huddled on the floor in the hallway outside my bedroom as I carefully opened the fire-safe box where I had been storing this letter along with the journals Bob had kept for Henry and Arthur.

Carefully I unfolded the piece of paper and gently pulled at the frayed pieces left from where I had ripped it from the spiral notebook. Taking a deep breath, I put my hand to my heart, trying to calm its frantic activity.

> Dear Irene,   March-
>
>   I want to write you letters. I feel like I've done a
> pretty good job being open and honest throughout
> this whole lymphoma thing with some exceptions,
> for what were probably selfish reasons. So this is not
> really just about the lymphoma. It's really just about
> me wanting to write you letters.

You are the most wonderful person in my life. I know you probably get sick of me writing this but I can't believe my luck at getting to share lives with you.

Most of this will probably just be blibber-blabber, some of it might be scribble-scrabble ...

Bob's handwriting became illegible and then turned to scratches on the paper, then ... nothing. I visualized Bob sitting in a blue fake leather recliner with an IV in his arm, slowly dripping the chemo into his blood system. The notebook sat in his lap, and he had a pen in his hand, poised to write. But his hand was not moving. His eyes were glassy. His heavily lashed eyelids drooped, and his head sagged forward.

"That's it?" I asked, incredulous, coming back to the present moment. "I waited a year for this?"

My heart was now immobile in my chest, and I wanted to laugh at the same time. This moment was so "Irene and Bob" that I could hardly stand it. I'd planned and planned, and Bob had gotten his understated point across with perfect clarity. You can't plan everything. You have to relish the tiny moments and implied affections, the hawk sightings and the subtle gestures and comforts of everyday life.

Bob had made no deathbed confessions. And now, a year later, he wasn't going to supply me with endearments from beyond the grave. His feelings for me had to be taken at face value. They were what they were when they were, and that was enough.

CHAPTER SEVEN

Dog Mountain

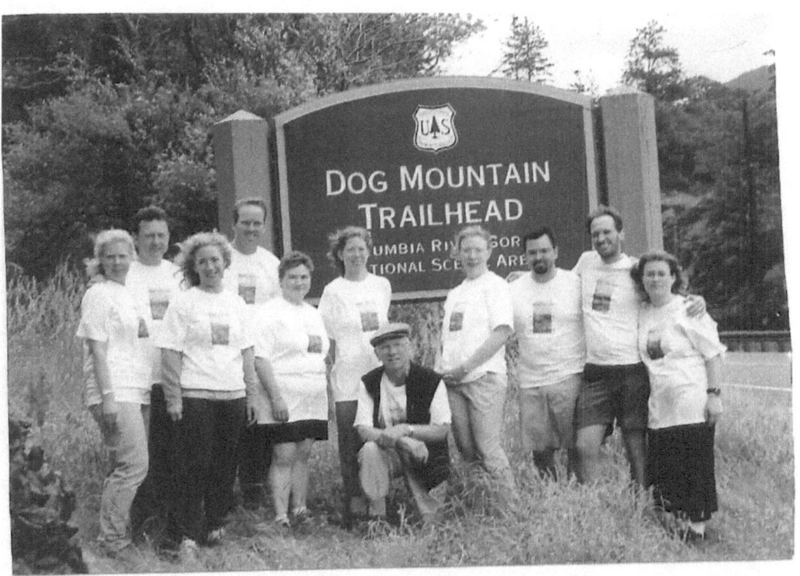

Happiness is a journey,
not a destination.
Souza

Blue balloons with yellow butterflies on them floated above the dining room table, tethered by curly ribbons. One big purple balloon with "Forever 39" across it stood out among all the fluttering wings. From the kitchen I heard the distinct rustling of the cellophane being gnawed, followed shortly by the lovely sound of the cat hacking up the ribbon he had just eaten.

For Bob's birthday, I had decided to tackle pizza making, a task I had yet to undertake since his death. I dragged the Kitchen Aid out from the back of the cabinet where it was hiding behind the cereal boxes. Dusting it off, I felt so guilty. The Kitchen Aid had once held a spot of such prominence in our kitchen and was now relegated to the dark depths of a cabinet. I was just hoping that Bob's sisters would be able to tell me about all the different parts.

Next I had to find the recipe he used for the crust. Thumbing through his cookbooks, I could picture Bob's focused gaze as he paged through them on a Saturday morning, hoping to become inspired. I was startled out of my reverie when a Post-it note drifted out of the Better Homes and Gardens cookbook that held the coveted pizza crust recipe.

I expected to find Bob's doodling of his own version of a recipe. He often played with the measurements in a very scientific way; "¼ cup" and "½ teaspoon" with a big "??" were often found in the margins of his favorite recipes.

Irene

Do whatever, Be comfortable, Breathe Deep and Enjoy Life.
I'll be back shortly.

Bob

My breath came a little shorter. The note felt like a message from beyond. When did Bob write this? It was early enough in our relationship that he was still calling me Irene. We must have still been living separately since he was telling me to be comfortable. This note must have been marking a page in this cookbook for years. Bob had probably pulled the note off the top one day, in a hurry to mark the recipe in question. How many times had Bob opened up this book and moved this tiny piece of paper and held it between his finger and thumb while he read the recipe? Touching the note, for an instant I could feel his fingertips on mine, a gentle graze.

Later, after all the Kitchen Aid parts had been washed, the four pizzas eaten, and the frosting from the apple pastry dessert had been licked from our fingers, the group all went out to the front yard and sent the balloons off into the universe. Ten of us watched as the balloons drifted into the clouds and become little bitty dots against the blue sky.

As I stood there in the brisk wind and squinted into the sun, I could feel my hawk tattoo pulse a little as the skin stitched itself back together over the bird with its wings spread out in flight. I thought about that note from Bob.

"Enjoy Life", he had told me.

≈≈

Lori and Derek, up from Chicago, came to visit. Bob and I met Lori soon after moving to Portland. She and her then-boyfriend walked into a meditation workshop we were attending. Her long, brown, curly hair framed a thin oval face that could barely contain her smile. When they introduced themselves to the group, they said they had just moved to Portland from Illinois. All fellow Midwesterners, we became friends.

The three of us eventually returned to our roots and remained in contact. (I take full credit for introducing Lori and Derek. His mom, who was also my boss, was equally involved, but I like to leave that part out.) Some people say a crisis like losing your spouse can make or break a friendship. The three of us seemed to flourish in my new situation. I could always rely on them to listen and offer well-thought-out, honest advice. They were never short on encouragement.

During the nickel tour of my house, Lori lingered in front of my full-length mirror upstairs in the hallway.

Courage
Patience
Resilience
Perseverance
Capacity to Distance
Sense of Humor

From now on I want to …

These affirmations were posted at the top of the mirror and on every other mirror of the house as well as on my refrigerator.

"Tell me about these," Lori said in that social worker/leading question way.

"A friend sent me a book called *The Courage to Grieve*, by Judy Tatelbaum, for the first anniversary of Bob's death," I answered. The friend had become a young widow ten years earlier and felt the book helped her enormously.

"These are the skills a person needs to get through grief. They remind me what I should be focused on," I explained. "I need to look forward, not back. What do I want for my life now, as opposed to what I wanted for it when Bob was alive?"

Grief was like an enormous sand dune, and getting over it involved two steps forward and one and a half steps back. This sand beneath my feet was constantly moving, always threatening a slide back down to the bottom. But I just kept doggedly marching up the dune, one foot in front of the other. Reading this list every day strengthened me and gave me hope. The list reminded me of what I had already accomplished and the strengths I already had. It hadn't been easy to get where I was now, but I had courage, and I would persevere. I was working on patience.

Look how far I had already come.

I was a warrior, a survivor.

Grieving—it's not for sissies.

≈≈

One late spring day at the assisted living facility where I worked, I pushed one of the participants at the day center in her wheelchair to her beauty shop appointment. I noticed a spry elderly lady in a blue cardigan sweater opening the door to her apartment. I noticed she had a hyphenated name above her door.

Hyphenated surnames are very unusual for someone of that generation, and I asked her about it as we passed by.

"I had two husbands, and I loved them both," she answered, looking up toward me as she jiggled her lock a bit. A broad, open smile spread across her face and lit her eyes with nostalgia.

Without warning, I started silently weeping right there in the middle of the hallway, and these were tears of joy. My hands gripped the wheelchair for balance. So much became clear in that moment, with that simple statement. People shuffled around me with their walkers and canes on their way to the dining room. I wondered if they could see the ray of light that must be surrounding me or feel the vibrating hum.

That was what I wanted my story to be.

I couldn't live my life feeling bitter. I didn't want to live with a chip on my shoulder, as if the world owed me something because my husband died. I couldn't go on feeling indignant and resentful. I wanted to look at this as an opportunity, an opportunity to take charge of my life and move in a different direction. I could love two good men in a lifetime. Not everyone has the chance to do that.

I felt my heart expanding in my chest. The Grinch must have felt the same way on top of that mountain on Christmas morning when he heard those Who's sing. This unsuspecting lady was my Who. I had to risk a broken heart again. I could do nothing else.

It would be far worse to have nothing worth a broken heart.

Having another relationship would do nothing to negate the relationship I had with Bob. I could love them both.

The heart's love is boundless.

≈≈

Every time I got into the car that spring, I recalled just how pathetic our last summer, the first summer after Bob died, had been. From the driver's seat, I would see the State Park stickers that lined the left side of the windshield. 2000, 2001, 2002, 2003, their colorful boxes lined up one on top of the other. These stickers were a sign of activity and nature, good living and fresh air.

But that rainbow stopped short at 2003. It was now April of 2005, and I had no 2004 sticker. That meant I had not had a reason, in the entire year of 2004, to purchase a State Park sticker. No good living and fresh air for an entire year?

That had to change.

My neighbor, Matt, and I planned a bike-riding excursion with our kids. Matt was the perfect neighbor, friendly but not intrusive, always willing to help the neighbor widow out. I even found him cleaning my gutters one sunny fall afternoon. He had two young kids and was an expert in all issues related to bikes. He had graciously helped me out quite a few times already with basic maintenance on our bikes and guidance with the trailer and bike rack. He seemed to appreciate Bob's Italian road bike from the 1970s that I had hung in the garage, hoping the boys might become interested in it one day.

Matt was taking us along the Glacial Drumlin Trail in Lake Country, as he called it, just west of Milwaukee. I had never been on this trail. I was grateful to have the motivation and the help to get out on our first biking excursion without Bob. For my mental health I needed the three of us to get back out on our bikes, and I figured I just had to make it through the first trip.

Unfortunately, that did not happen on this trip. About five feet away from the car, my tire blew out (due to inactivity, I am sure!) and we had to improvise some new plans. We ended up at the tower in a state park nearby where the kids could run around a bit and climb the tower.

"Well, at least we got you a state park sticker today," Matt said as we watched the children collect sticks on the hill.

I nodded vigorously; I felt such a surge of power and happiness about that darn state park sticker. My eyes watered when I snatched it out of the poor innocent state park worker's hand, and my heart skipped a few beats when I saw the picture of the hawk on the sticker. As I peeled the back and carefully spread that beautiful bird smoothly on my windshield, I smiled toward the sky. I know Bob was looking on and cheering for me.

2005, it said in yellow numbers. The three of us were on our way; no matter what happened now at least I had proof that in 2005 I had at least one day of sunshine and good living.

≈≈

The trip to Dog Mountain to scatter Bob's ashes was coming up quickly, and preparations grew fast and furious. When I thought of the idea back after he first died, this journey seemed so far away. Now flights were being booked, hotel rooms were being reserved, T-shirts were being designed, and I was in major training. I was in nothing like the physical condition I'd had when we were living out in Portland, and I didn't want to struggle up the mountain when I was supposed to be the leader of the pack.

At every chance, I walked in the park near my house. It had two sets of stairs, and I walked up and down those two flights over and over again; it was the only way to get any elevation. Several times, while marching up and down, I saw a hawk gliding above the canopy of trees. Once it perched on a branch and looked down at me. It must have been the same one I had seen that first time from the playground; this area was part of that same park. I thought of these sightings as messages from Bob, encouragement to keep climbing, get up that mountain, and put him where he belonged.

The night before we left for Oregon, my dad helped me transfer Bob's ashes from the urn into a plastic bag for the flight and then the hike. I had a vision of dumping the ashes directly from the urn onto the mountain; that seemed more poetic somehow. But practically I knew there was no way to get the thirty-pound marble urn up that mountain. So I carefully separated Bob's remains into three different baggies—one for the mountain, one for Henry, and one for Arthur in case they ever wanted to scatter them somewhere when they got older.

As I slowly poured the contents into the Ziploc bag my dad held, I was grateful that my sister, Teri, had warned me about the texture of the ashes. It would have been a shock to discover the chunks of bone as I poured them from one bag to another instead of the fine powder one expects after viewing scenes involving human ashes on TV shows and movies.

≈≈

Finally on the plane, I sat next to my dad as Arthur slept and Henry busied himself with a sticker book. Somehow my dad and I began discussing what I might be looking for in my next husband. An odd topic considering the reason for our current trip, but my dad took this conversation very seriously. He started a list: age 35–50, employed, likes to travel, good with children were the first few items.

Tentatively I mentioned a conversation about dating with some girlfriends. The three ladies and I were sitting in my backyard, and our six children hung in various positions from my white cedar play structure. The wood chips I had just poured around the structure still looked neat and clean.

I had confessed my latest obsession, the waste of my sexual prime. Truly I was aghast at the unfairness of being shut down just as I should have been hitting my stride. I had been having fantasies of one-night stands and friends with benefits. Of course, I hadn't been successful with these endeavors when I was young and carefree, so the prospect of acting on these fantasies with two young boys and a home to run seemed more than remote.

I felt so ahead of the life curve. I developed a theory that the 35–45 decade was the make-or-break decade for marriages. Couples were either going to settle into a comfortable groove for the long haul or decide they needed to take another direction in life. As we got older, illness would become more common as well. Where did this theory leave me? Waiting around for people to divorce or die? That sounded awful.

I was always ahead of my time. Maybe I would be able to show other people the way.

That afternoon my friend, Christine, after listening to my tale of sexual woe, had mentioned a man from our church. He would be good to know and fun to hang out with, she said. Mike Hogan was his name. She knew he was divorced, and she had met him on the church camping trip. She would check out his situation for me, I told my dad. I might meet him when Henry and I went camping with the church in June.

Thinking highly of Christine, my dad absorbed this bit of information, nodding and stroking his chin while considering the possibilities. He leaned back in his chair and set his pen down on the legal pad where he had begun the list, as if our task were finished. I laughed. I knew a big part of their moving back to Milwaukee was to make sure I was "taken care of". To my dad, that probably meant getting me married off again.

≈≈

So there I stood, at the foot of the 3000-foot climb up Dog Mountain, with six family members and four friends surrounding me at the trailhead. The day I had been planning for the last sixteen months and trained for over the last two had arrived. I had tortured myself with a Kettlebell and done more repetitive stair climbing in the park then I cared to remember.

In my backpack I had eleven T-shirts of various sizes that stated, "I hiked 'The Dog' in honor of Bob Wellenstein 5/31/05". In with the T-shirts and water and snacks and rain gear was Bob, whom I'd successfully transported through airport security checks with death certificate in hand in case there was any question about the contents of the bag I hauled.

We started up the hill. I glanced up to the sky above the trailhead, hoping to glimpse a hawk, and there he was, just as I expected, circling the parking lot, observing, lending silent support. The wind whipped my damp hair across my face, and I shivered under my raincoat. It was just the kind of rainy, cool Pacific Northwest day Bob would have loved.

About a third of the way up, still enduring the switchbacks, my dad turned around. Due to some health problems, he decided it would be best if he waited down at the parking lot for us. As he passed me on the trail, he touched my backpack lightly.

"Bye, Bob, God speed," he said.

That simple gesture felt like an open-hand smack in the face. The reason for this event became clear. All the preparation had not been simply for a lovely hike, a nice gathering of likeminded folks.

My husband was to be spread at the top of this mountain. I was going to leave him here among the wildflowers. My heart began to race, and it was not from the exertion of the climb. After all the planning and anticipation that had gone into this day, I was scared I wouldn't be able to release him.

Could I really pour Bob out at the top of this mountain and walk away? Remembering my reaction when I had first tried leaving our wedding bands on the counter at the jeweler, I started to get more than a little nervous. Back before Christmas, Sarah and I had gone to her jeweler to have Bob's and my wedding bands made into a necklace. She and I stood at the counter and calmly discussed with the nice lady designer how the two rings would go together.

The jeweler picked the two white gold rings up and studied them while she spoke. "I want to be sure of what I am doing before I start to cut ..." she trailed off as if talking to herself. "If I just stacked them on top of each other, they would look like a snowman, but if I inserted one in the other, they would look more like a figure eight," she continued.

"The symbol of infinity," I interjected, excited about that idea.

The curly-haired jeweler then placed the rings on the counter to start the paperwork, still mumbling about the importance of her skill once the cutting started. I stared at those two silver circles, symbols of Bob's and my unending love, and all I could hear was "cut". Once she started the "cutting", she put it—as if she were saying that one word through a microphone. The rings looked so delicate and helpless laying there on the glass counter, and my ring finger felt oddly empty as my thumb reflexively moved to twirl the ring I was not wearing. Without realizing what I was doing I reached for the rings and scooped them off the counter, as if snatching the last cookie on the plate.

Startled, the jeweler looked up; her ringlets shook a bit.

"I can't do it," I said, with a catch in my throat, as I quickly put the rings back on. (I had been wearing Bob's ring on my right thumb since the day he died.)

"It's ok." Sarah had spoken reassuringly, placing her hand over mine. "We'll come back when you're ready."

Now, six months later, I fingered the necklace as I continued my trek up the mountain. I imagined myself standing frozen at the top, turning to everyone and saying, "Well, folks, thanks for coming. How about the same time next year?"

Had I dragged all these people out here and up this mountain in this crappy weather for nothing?

Bob and I had never discussed spreading his ashes on Dog Mountain. This was all my idea. I felt that Dog Mountain was where he belonged; it was the right place. His spirit could be anywhere it wanted to be in the universe, his body would forever be on Dog Mountain, in the part of the country he most loved, where he felt most himself, where we were at our best. He belonged there. He belonged among the wildflowers.

I knew this was true, but could I really do it?

Unaware of my misgivings, the group continued up the trail. We passed sword and maidenhair ferns that had slowly unfolded in the shaded hills and now stood at attention in big leafy clumps like enormous bunches of lettuce. The yellow Indian paintbrush that blanketed the windswept mountain looked just as bright as I remembered, even more so against the steel-gray sky. The delicate blue lupine seemed undaunted by the unrelenting wind.

The group made the steep three-mile ascent rather quickly, though not without some difficulty. A crippling fear of heights and rheumatoid arthritis were just two challenges people overcame that day to get to the top of the Dog.

I remembered the first time Bob and I hiked Dog Mountain. It was our first spring in Portland and Bob's birthday. We were still learning the ins and outs of the hiking scene in the Pacific Northwest. Bob had read about this hike in one of our hiking books that we would study over when planning our weekend jaunts. It was described as follows.

> The most spectacular wildflower meadows of the entire Columbia River Gorge drape the alp-like slopes of Dog Mountain. In May and June these hills are alive with the colors of Indian paintbrush and lupine. Even flowerless seasons provide breathtaking views of the Columbia Gorge. Such beauty has made the Dog Mountain Trail very popular. But it is not an easy hike, for the trail is challengingly steep throughout.
>
> William Sullivan, *100 Hikes in Northwest Oregon*

Bob's birthday is April 2. But never mind, it was his birthday, and the book does say that even off season, there are beautiful views. So off we went early that Saturday morning. We had the trail to ourselves, which was a good thing, because we wouldn't have wanted anyone else to witness my less-than-attractive efforts at getting up the hill that day. It is a wonder Bob ever wanted me to hike with him again.

I grumbled, I whined, I told him I couldn't make it when we got to the post stating that there was just .1 mile left to the summit. I was making myself miserable. Bob just silently, relentlessly, doggedly kept climbing, enjoying the view and the challenge as if a crazy woman was not beside him on the trail.

Bob was remarkably skilled at ignoring my little incidences and going about his business. I usually ended up thankful he had dragged me wherever it was that he had dragged me. On the way home, I would think about what we just saw and acknowledge how beautiful the gorge was, even without the flowers.

"Wow, that was really amazing, Bob! Gorgeous views of the gorge. Thanks for bringing me out here"

"Yup," he would respond simply before ceremoniously pointing out the window. "Hey, Renie, there's a hawk! You see that hawk?"

After that first experience with Dog Mountain it became my mission to get into better shape and enjoy that damn hike when those damn flowers were actually in bloom. Dog Mountain became an annual event for us during the remainder of our sojourn in Portland. We hiked it with different people, different dogs, in all sorts of different weather conditions, and even once when Bob was vomiting.

Without Bob, I would probably never have climbed Dog Mountain, opting to stay in bed and lounge about with coffee and a book and satisfying my need for fresh air with a walk in the funky neighborhood where we lived. Without Bob and his steady resilience in the face of my dramatic outbursts, I would have experienced a fraction of the gorgeous surroundings the Pacific Northwest has to offer, a fraction of what life has to offer. I was so lucky to have had him in my life and to have been part of his view of the world.

None of these people on this mountain today would be seeing this view if not for Bob. Otherwise, they may have never seen this part of the country, with its huge trees and lush ferns and this incredible river that was once so powerful that it carved a gorge between mountains and left waterfalls in its wake. We were all lucky to have a chance to experience this yellow mountainside; it was almost enough for me to believe in God.

≈≈

Once at the top, we searched for a dry place to sit and eat, but there was none. The drippy, cold wetness was inescapable. We gathered around some old logs protected by some trees and shivered while we ate. I felt that we had the place to ourselves. There was some small talk and the chaos of people following the distribution of the T-shirts, folks putting them on, lunging for the correct size, holding them up, and checking them out.

I knew people were waiting for me to act, and I felt that I should say something. I was so ready *not* to be the center of attention any more, to have nothing to say that anyone would want to hear. Being so close to tragedy makes everything a person says so profound.

I wanted to thank everyone for coming on this journey with me, and not just the hike. I wanted to tell them how much it meant to me to have them all here, what an incredible tribute their presence was to Bob and who he was, who we were. I wanted to tell them what I had learned through his death and the time after it and how each one and countless others had helped me. I wanted to explain why I wanted Bob on Dog Mountain and why I wanted the song "Wildflowers" by Tom Petty played while I scattered him here.

I could say hardly a word. Instead I muttered something like, "I think the song speaks for itself."

Following my lead, everyone stood up, and people formed a U around me, and the music began, "You belong, among the wild flowers", the wind drowned out much of it, but the meaning was still there.

Just when I began to walk forward, a woman materialized out of the mist, dressed in full Pacific Northwest hiking gear complete with a hat and carrying a walking stick. Not recognizing the oddity of a group of ten people on a rainy weekday, all wearing the same shirts, with one standing in the middle and holding a bag full of suspicious material, the woman barreled forward and asked, "Have you seen a dog? Have you seen my dog?"

We all just stood there, mute, shaking our heads in mutual agreement. No, we hadn't seen any dog. She walked back into the mist, continuing her search.

We started over. I hesitated only a moment before pitching forward, opening the bag, and throwing Bob into the wind, among the wildflowers.

The wind was blowing hard, and I had considered how I should go about this scattering business so as not to have the ashes blow back into my face as ashes might in some made-for-TV movie. My plans were thwarted. Bob's last lesson to me was that you can't plan everything. Back he came toward me in the swirling wind. *Plop*, some of him landed on my hiking boots. Without thinking, I turned around and yelled to the group, "He's all over my boots! Bob's on my boots."

Just at that moment, the clouds broke open, and for about thirty seconds, we could see the smooth water of the Columbia River Gorge down below and the rocky hills of Oregon jutting up on the other side.

≈≈

Intellectually I knew these ashes were not Bob, just the remains of the vessel Bob used in this life. But I am sentimental, and those ashes meant something to me. I missed Bob's physical body as much as his presence and his energy. I missed Bob and everything those three letters meant. I missed who I was when I was with him and the activities we did because we were together. The people we knew, the places we went, the way I viewed the world when I was with him—I missed all these. Bob made me a better person. I always felt so safe with Bob, as if everything would be OK and somehow taken care of.

I threw all that weight away, scattered the ashes of Bob and our life together to the wind and the flowers, and walked down that mountain by myself. I never imagined that departure would feel the way it did—as if I were abandoning him, walking away from our life together.

I felt irritated with my friends and family as they began their idle chatter while we descended.

Do you understand what just happened here, people? I wanted to scream that I didn't care what just happened on the last episode of *Everybody Loves Raymond*. I just left my husband. I just walked away from my life, my past.

Despite myself, however, I was walking into my future.

The physical work of walking down that mountain meant more for me in my recovery than anything else I had done for myself since Bob was first diagnosed. A miraculous change began as I continued my descent. I felt lighter with every step, letting go of the burden of the physical part of a person, all that humanness and complexity that keeps people with us on this Earth.

I wanted to live for the future and in the present, but I couldn't just abandon the past. People told me I had to move on, but I felt that I could move *forward*, a subtle yet distinct difference. Yes, I had just parted with Bob physically, but his spirit remained with me. I could still feel his spirit and take him with me, being neither weighed down nor held back.

I had discovered a well-kept secret; our relationship was not over, but had just changed shape. I got to take the best of Bob with me and incorporate him into who I was now. I could still be that better person.

Bob was where he belonged now, and so was I.

Did I hope for closure? Does closing a door mean you can never open it again and look in? Or does it mean that you have to shut the door and not bring anything with you from that room into the new one? Can people wander in and out of rooms? Do people moving into new homes not take any mementos with them from their former lives?

What did I hope for? I hoped for peace, I hoped for relief, I hoped for strength, I hoped to move forward, I hoped to bring Bob's spirit with me, I hoped that I had learned something from this experience, and I hoped that he hadn't died for nothing. I hoped for happiness. I hoped for hope itself.

≈≈

Bob's ashes remained on my hiking boots for the rest of that trip through the Northwest. Every hike we went on, I would stomp my boot a little and stomp some of Bob out onto the trail, meanwhile thinking how appropriate it was that Bob would be shaken out onto a trail in the Olympic National Forest right next to a banana slug.

How funny I must have looked to an observer, a mom hiking along a trail with a toddler in a carrier on her back and a four-year-old running ahead to hide in the enormous felled logs. And periodically the mom would stop and stomp her foot on the trail, smiling to herself as she glanced toward the top of the trees for a hawk, quietly observing.

Bob would have grinned at the image.

Chapter Eight

Glow

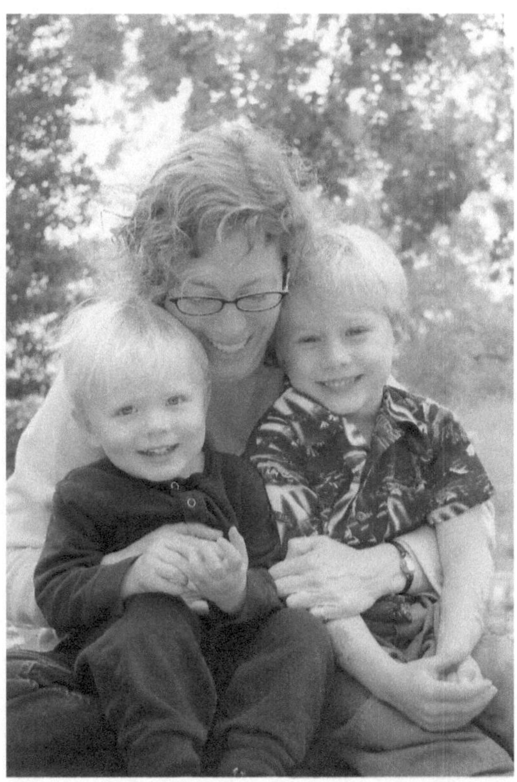

Let us continue now this joyous task of living.
Author unknown

≈≈

Tom Petty was blasting on my boom box outside the bathroom, and I was singing at the top of my lungs, "….You don't know what it's like, to be meeeeeee…" as I bopped in front of the mirror and got ready for a night out with my girlfriend, Jeanne. We were only going to see a movie, but I relished the fact that I was currently alone in my house. I was looking forward to going out and then coming home to a quiet house where everything was in its place and waking up the next morning with no one staring at me asking to see my feet.

Looking at myself in the mirror, as I had so many times in the past two years, I realized I was no longer wondering what people saw when they looked at me. I wasn't hiding anything anymore. I wasn't pretending to live while just going through the motions. My face had definition again. I felt free.

Turning sideways toward the full-length mirror, I admired my new outfit. I had finally bought myself some new clothes, and they were colorful. I was tired of looking like a bag lady in beige.

"Thirty-seven and wearing tighter shirts" was my new motto, borrowed from a friend in Portland. I added "wearing foundation" to that motto as well. I had never worn makeup, and the results weren't bad.

I looked good! I felt good!

The CD switched to Peter Himmelman "…..Imperfect world, I miss your laugh and your perfect face…", and I kept singing at the top of my lungs, swinging my hips in those tight-fitting jeans.

≈≈

"Hey, Mommy, I've got an idea." Henry came around the corner from the dining room and stood in front of the microwave. His eyes flashed with excitement, and his voice was high.

"Oh yeah? What is it, buddy?" I asked, turning my attention from the dishes to his wide smile. Rarely did I get such open expression from him. This had to be good.

"You could go get us a new daddy!"

He stood in front of me, his hair white already from the sun and his eyes as blue as a cloudless summer day, his expression as exuberant as if he had just discovered the recipe for world peace … and expectant, as if I could just run down to the local store where they were having a sale on daddies.

I needed that word for laughter mixed with tears again.

≈≈

I actually had a great time last night. The thought struck me as I stood in line at the co-op grocery store. Was that easy laughter and conversation around the dinner table last night with Jeanne and Jim? Just like old times. When I told them about Henry learning to ride his bicycle in front of the entire block (he did it on the first try), I was so proud. Not only because he did such an awesome job but because the event had not been bittersweet. It was all sweet as I watched Henry's determined face fly past me on the sidewalk, full of power and freedom and possibility.

Standing there patiently, watching the person in front of me unload her cart, I became acutely aware of how good it felt to live in my body at that moment. I felt well-fed and lean, and my skin felt warm and smelled like fresh grass from a summer of outdoor activities. Taking my dried mangos and red pepper out of my basket, I was mindful of how the rich orange and red looked against each other.

The thought of the tangy sweetness of the red pepper reminded me how far I had come from the days of instant oatmeal for dinner every night. I had continued to enjoy my five favorites of Bob's recipes and had found a few of my own that the three of us could enjoy. The house felt a bit richer now. Henry and I had even managed the pancake recipe a few times—no more Bisquick for us.

We had been in the new house a year and experienced each season there. It had been quite a summer. I had successfully checked off the last events on my list of accomplishments I needed to perform before I could officially check "grieving" off my to-do list.

After the scattering of Bob's ashes, I had determined there were only two more major activities to figure out on my own before I could feel confident that the three of us would carry on without Bob in a manner that I could live with. These activities were camping and biking.

My lips curled up a bit as I remembered a camping trip that Henry and I took with the church. I had to ask my neighbor to help me properly attach the bike rack to the car, but we made it there and got the tent up and a fire going. We had only hot dogs to cook over the fire, but that was OK. We two had camped "Irene McGoldrick style". None of the gourmet camping that Bob liked to do for us—I had brought a box of Total cereal and some Pop Tarts that we ate straight out of the box.

Then there was the afternoon I successfully mounted the bike rack on the back of the Subaru all by myself and the three of us were off on a biking adventure along our new favorite trail. It was hot, and I could smell a bit of drying hay and manure in the air from the nearby farms. We looked like any family out for a Sunday ride, enjoying the beautiful afternoon. I had no "W" stamped on my forehead; no one knew the obstacles I had overcome to be out there that day. We were just a mom with one child in the trailer in the back and the other child peddling furiously with his short legs to keep up.

Lost in my musings, I had completely forgotten that I was at the grocery store and was startled when Les, the friendly checker who always remembered my member number, spoke.

"You've got your glow back," he said.

My face flushed and my smile was sincere in reaction to the compliment.

≈≈

All summer I had known that on August 24, I had religious education training at church. All summer I had known that Mike Hogan would be attending this meeting. Mike was the man I had mentioned to my dad on the plane to Oregon to scatter Bob's ashes. He came highly recommended as someone with whom I could "get back out there".

I was very interested in getting back out there. I didn't see myself alone for the long haul, so I needed to get back out there. But dating?

My friends seemed a bit too anxious to live vicariously through any possible dating debâcle. While I honestly felt ready to meet someone, the idea of actually dating made me feel like a cold hand was squeezing my stomach. Some friends in Chicago mentioned a prospective suitor and even had a plan for us to meet. The mere idea that this meeting could really happen sent me into a small-scale panic attack, actually forcing me to clutch my chest while I cradled the phone to my ear for the happy set-up chatter on the other end.

The next day I took the boys to a lake with Sarah and her daughter, Clara, and I was telling her about my anxiety at the idea of a date.

"Interesting," Sarah said thoughtfully as we watched the kids dig in the wet sand. "Jeff (the house clearing/medium guy) asked about you yesterday, and I told him you were feeling ready to date but that nothing was going on in that regard yet. His response was that there was a person circling and that you just have to let go of your apprehension."

Goosebumps rose on my arms even out in the hot sun. Was the secret speaking again? Was this voice my destiny? Was it my higher self, and had it been talking to me all along?

While I was busy figuring out bike racks and camping menus and dealing with sexual frustration and anxiety, I had August 24th in my mind like the period at the end of a sentence. It was a little something to look forward to, a ray of sunshine breaking through the clouds. But it had always been in the future, and now the date was here.

Arriving late at the training, I stood in the back and looked around the room and wondered which man was Mike Hogan. My eyes rested on each man in the room; some I recognized, but most I didn't.

My eyes lingered on a man with graying sideburns and thick, wavy hair that begged for hands to be run through it. I noticed his bold glasses and that he was not much taller than me. He had on long shorts and leather sandals and had that slightly preppy look that I enjoy in men. Standing with his arms across his chest and his papers crumpled in one hand, he leaned to one side and appeared slightly bewildered by the situation, as if unsure that he was in the right place.

I hope that's him. I noted his engaging manner with the people in his group. As he breezed by me on the way to the classrooms, I caught a glimpse of his name tag—"Mike H ..." something. *Now what?*

Since attempting eye contact with this wavy-haired gentleman when we passed each other in the hallway hadn't had the desired effect (i.e., he would immediately be blown over by my brilliance and ask me on a date that instant) I found myself lurking by the brochures during the social hour after the training, pretending to read about what Jesus had said about homosexuals while I waited for him to be alone so I could introduce myself.

This was no easy task; he was a very social guy. Each time I glanced his way, he was talking animatedly to someone. His arms were fully engaged with his conversation, and he laughed easily. His eyes darted around the room as if he didn't want to miss an opportunity to talk to someone else.

Every cell in my body wanted to walk out of that room, run down the dark hallway past the stained glass that surrounded the sanctuary, leap in my car, and return to the safety of my empty home. No one would ever have to know. My heart pounded, and I chastised myself for being pathetic. I couldn't even introduce myself to a man at a church gathering. This inability did not bode well for any potential dating activity in my future.

If this man had been Bob, he and I would have met at the brochure rack, both aimlessly loitering in the corners while hiding from the crowd. Finally, however, this man was alone, and I walked briskly toward him before I could head for the door instead.

"Are you Mike Hogan?" I asked, cocking my head to one side and trying to sound casual, still clutching the crinkled and now damp brochure in my hand.

"I am," he responded, looking down at his name tag as if checking to be sure.

"You know Christine Wolf?" I stammered, still trying to sound casual.

"So, what's your story?" Mike asked me with a wave of his hand after we had exhausted the initial small talk about our mutual friend.

"Ummm ... well," I began. How does one answer that? I wanted him to know I was single, but how was I to do that gracefully? He didn't really want the whole gruesome story, I was sure of that, but after mentioning the boys and my work, I was convinced that he thought my husband was at home with the children. I was thankful that Mike kept right on talking while my brain went into overdrive for some graceful way to let him know my situation.

"Well, my ex ..." he began, the slightest frustration creeping into his voice. And there was my opening.

"That's why it's better to be widowed," I interjected. I then proceeded to turn ten shades of red after hearing the words come out of my mouth—not my most graceful introductory move with a stranger. Well, at least he now knew I was single—single and crazy, perhaps, but single.

Luckily for me, Mike handled the situation with far more poise and acted as if my admission was the most normal remark in the world when meeting someone for the first time at a church event. He must have found the circumstances somewhat endearing because he did ask me to have coffee or wine with him after we closed the social hour. I chose wine.

Far more relaxed after a glass of wine at the Irish pub near the church, we continued our banter. I felt surprisingly natural despite being on my first date in twelve years, if a date was what we could call this little adventure.

Mike offered to walk me to my car after we left the pub, but as we approached the car, he suddenly decided he was not ready for the evening to end yet and asked if I was interested in a walk by the lake.

Just wait until my girlfriends heard about this!

"Can I hold your hand?" Mike asked as we walked along the lakefront. The moon reflected on the water and cast little dots of light that shimmered on the tiny waves.

"Ssssure." I hoped to sound more confident than I felt. He grabbed my hand with confidence; his grip felt strong and protective. I was intensely aware of how different this hand was from the hand I was used to holding.

I'm holding another man's hand. It feels smaller, fleshier, a bit rougher and stronger. Bob had slender fingers and smooth palms, and when I held his hand, I could feel a gentle, grounding force slide up my arm and surround me, as if he just wanted to exist beside me. This hand felt bolder and firmer, and this man's pace was quicker, as if he wanted to lead me somewhere.

We eventually made it back to my car, where Mike took my face in those strong hands, looked me in the eyes, and kissed me assuredly three times before I could think any *will he, won't he, should we, shouldn't we* thoughts.

"I'll call you tomorrow," he said, and held the car door open for me.

Turning blindly toward the car, I somehow managed to get in and turn the key. I couldn't begin to process what another man's lips felt like; I was still too busy obsessing about the hand. Driving the city streets toward home, my hand to my chest, inhaling deeply, trying to get my heart steadied, I attempted to keep my eyes on the road and the street lights.

I felt a presence in the car, a slight touch to the shoulder. Was that just a slender, smooth hand I felt, a gentle nudge?

"Well, Bob, I guess you saw all that," I said out loud in the car. "I just kissed another man ... and I kinda liked it ... That's OK, right? Yeah, it's OK, it's OK." I answered my own question. "Oh, my God, that was just the most romantic night of my life … is that bad to say? What does that mean? It's so weird, Bob, so weird." I began to babble, my heart racing now. Was it from excitement, fear, attraction, or all of the above?

Somehow making it home and into my bedroom, I racked my brain for someone to call at this late hour. I could not wait until morning to share the news of this unexpected evening. Coming up with no one, I flopped back on the bed, hand to forehead in disbelief, and my heart still pounding, a giddy smile across my face while I reviewed the events of the night.

I wonder if he'll call? He seemed sincere. He'll call … I'm sure … I think. Even if Mike Hogan never calls, at least I had a great first date in this new life of mine. Right?

"Right, Bob?" I said aloud, aware how nutty this situation was. I was talking to an empty room.

"Renie, don't worry," I sighed, answering myself.

Plan B

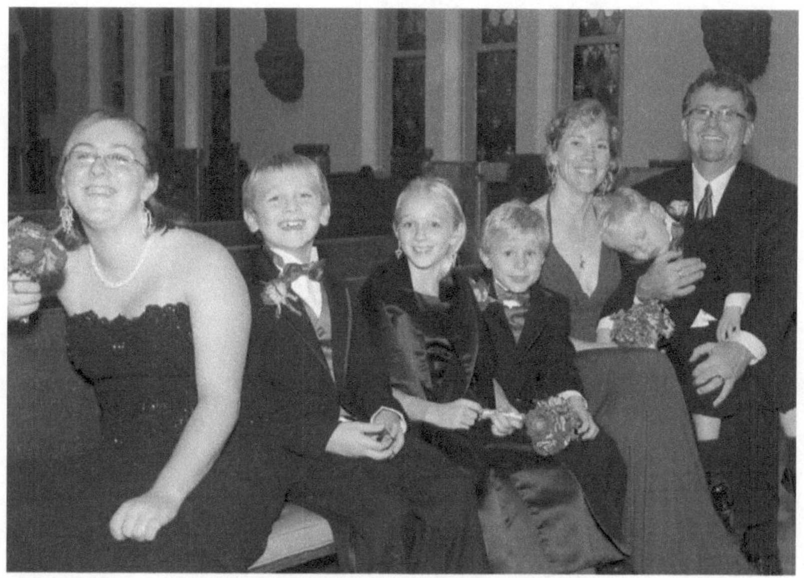

Hangovers come with love,
yet love's the cure for hangovers.
Mawlana Jalal-al-Din Rumi

On March 29, 2006, the second anniversary of Bob's death, I found myself on my back in the middle of the living room. I had my knees bent and my arms stretched out to each side as if making the top half of a snow angel. Pictures and cards from Bob's last week alive and the memorial lay around me, and Peter Himmelman blasted from the stereo.

Following my second chai of the day with Sarah, I felt the need to come home and play every song that reminded me of Bob. I just kept hitting "play again" when "Measure" came on, remembering how Bob loved to dance around the living room in our old house and sing it to me.

"You and I got a piece of that infinite thing," he had sung. He might play a little air guitar and close his eyes for effect.

The vibration under my back from the speakers felt like a little massage, and I could hear the pounding and heavy footsteps coming from the floor above me. The remodel of the upper portion of my bungalow had begun several weeks earlier because the house needed a little help to accommodate Mike and his three children.

Closing my eyes, I let the tears stream down my face, a waterfall of emotion. I was attempting to reconcile all the thoughts swirling in my head.

How can I miss Bob so much and be so excited about planning my wedding to Mike at the same time? How can I innocently plan for a wedding when I know, so vividly, how marriages can end? How can my situation feel so wrong and so right? How can I have moments of feeling the happiest I've ever felt when Bob is not here with me? Is my happiness in correlation with my sorrow? Since I have felt such deep sorrow, can I now experience greater joy?

Finally I surrendered to the all-too-memorable fetal position. I could feel the tears spread out against my skin against the wet carpet.

When Mike arrived home later that evening, my crying session might have never happened. All evidence had been packed away, and my eyes were dry—red and swollen maybe, but dry. Mike deftly avoided the subject, but his eyes showed their concern. Little wrinkles lined them, and their normal light blue color looked as gray as a cloud-covered ocean. He had been distant all week, still negotiating the best way to handle the waves of grief that splashed onto him now as well. His first instinct was to help me and protect me from the deluge. He was working hard on waiting out the storm.

The workmen had left, his kids were with their mom, and my boys were in bed, so the house was finally quiet. The two of us busied ourselves with the evening chores in the kitchen, avoiding eye contact as best we could. I was still getting used to Mike's energy in the house. He took up more space then I was used to giving over to a partner, and his thoughts were not contained like Bob's thoughts had been; they practically flashed neon.

It wasn't long before he spoke, his cadence quick, as if he might forget something if he took too long to express himself. "I just realized this past week that you'd rather be with Bob than me. I don't know what to do with that." He sat heavily onto the bench in the kitchen and leaned his square frame against the window. The darkening sky framed him, and I saw a few light stars dotting the horizon as I walked over to pull down the blinds.

The truth of his words stung like a slap.

"We can't use that word 'rather'," I said slowly and carefully. "It's a slippery slope. Of course, I would rather Bob wasn't dead and he was here raising his boys with me." Back at the sink I took a long, deep breath and closed my eyes to collect my thoughts. "But that's not the case. It just simply isn't so. It can't be." I paused between each word and continued to breathe, trying not to cry, focusing on the soapy dish in my hands.

Then I continued thoughtfully, the words forming in my head just a moment before they came out of my mouth. "You can't think of yourself as my second choice. You have to think of yourself as my first choice for this life, my new life, my new plan."

Then we both started laughing, laughing and crying, thinking of this crazy plan. At one time my plan was to never marry, to never have kids, now I would be twice married, have five kids. I could hear the collective laughter of all my friends and family, the irony of this situation too rich to pass up.

To marry a divorced man with three children—that was never part of the plan.

Plans change.

Acknowledgments

There are numerous people who have helped me along the way to make this book a reality. There were editor friends who had the courage to tell me when my sarcasm was not coming through on the page, family who encouraged me despite their concern of how they might be portrayed in the story and artist friends who donated their expertise to a self described technophobe. My early readers helped shape the final version of the book and became my friends along the way, a fact I find worth all the sacrifice it took to make this vision a reality.

I hesitate to start naming people for fear that I might forget someone. So, suffice it to say, to those who have helped and supported me along this entire journey, you know who you are, and I thank you, wholeheartedly. Special thanks to Jim Wieland, for the fabulous cover photo, the author photograph, and many of the interior shots. You can find his information on my website www.ms-dh.com.

Specifically, I would like to thank Bob, for giving me a story worth telling, Mike, for giving me the space and courage to tell it, and Henry and Arthur for reminding me every day of a wonderful man who, too briefly, walked among us.